# WHERE DO DOCTORS
# HIDE THEIR WINGS?

# WHERE DO DOCTORS HIDE THEIR WINGS?

Dennis G. McKenna, PA-C

**READS.**

Marietta, Georgia

WHERE DO DOCTORS HIDE THEIR WINGS

By Dennis G. McKenna, PAC

Copyright 2010, 2013

Published by PM Reads, a division of McKenna Project
Marietta, Georgia

Library of Congress Control Number: 2013910938

ISBN 978-0-9891593-0-2

I HAVE KNOWN DENNY MCKENNA for many years and not long ago I needed a physician referral. He said, "you must see Dr. G -he has wings." When I arrived for my appointment I said, " Denny McKenna said You have wings", He smiled and said, "If Denny said that I will do my best." Now I understand exactly what the statement means. Fascinating read from start to finish. I could not put the book down. A moving story painted with words you will never forget! I was there with your every move. You painted the picture in living motion of each event. I felt I was beside you, seeing, smelling, and feeling every-thing as it happened. I smelled the smoke and heard the water drip from the Dr.'s pocket as you put out the fire! I saw you run across the street retrieving the wine and the Dr. counting his change. And I saw the smile on your face when the patient walked out of the hospital. A must read for everyone! Thank you Denny for letting us peak into a corner of your world. We are waiting for more!

*Phyllis Slaght, Health Care Consultant*


THANKS FOR SHARING. CHOKED ME up a bit cause some of the stories are just too real and still hurt after many years. But I guess that's good. Denny's observation of the quiet of the veteran patient is the first thing that struck me when reading his book as it is a remark-able observation for someone who has not served in the military – especially in a combat zone. There is no need for these warriors to discuss experiences or the injuries that brought them to the VA for help – they know them even if they have not experienced them. This unstated awareness and tightness of the military family, the military base and the military unit are impossible to describe to a civilian but Denny has felt it and I expect other providers in the VA system have as well. These wounded patriots signed up for duty that they knew might cost them their lives. They are just looking for someone to show them the same care that they showed for our country and fortunately there are many really caring staff in the VA system.

*William (Bill) Paraska*
*Colonel, USAF (Retired)*

IN MY 30 YEAR NURSING career, I have worked with many physicians and it has been my experience that some not only have wings but also seem to have a magic wand. Gifted women and men with an emotional involvement with their patients and a sincere love of humanity is a powerful combination. As we go dancing through life with an occasional fall, some more graceful than others, it is reassuring to know that there are people that have dedicated their lives to helping us "get back up again". This book reminds you that these people exist.

*Barbara Anderson RN*

DEDICATION:

# How It All Began

I AM PERMANENTLY INDEBTED TO these physicians who gave tirelessly to my education. Their generous tutelage over the decades fueled my pursuit of the art and science of medicine. They taught me to love their craft and continually hunger for ever-expanding depths of knowledge.

It was at their side that I grew to love my patients as persons. They taught me how to gently distinguish the person from the malady, honoring the best in each of them so that they may, in turn, contribute to others.

Medicine, I came to discover, is an art of restoring health, dignity and value to all humanity. The laying on of hands to assess one's ills has a function of discovery and diagnostic value, but it is also an imparting of energy from the practitioner to the patient.

Physicians never discuss these phenomena as one avoids the implication that healing is in some manner a super-natural phenomenon. But, as intimately as I have known them in their pursuits on behalf of their patients, I can unapologetically state that this is so with startling frequency.

It is, in fact, my reason for writing this book and the impetus for this conversation.

# Acknowledgements

First and foremost, my thanks and gratitude goes to my loving family: My wife Peg and our two children, our daughter, Shannon and son, Joseph for their sacrifices and support of my work, often at the expense of their own needs.

I am also forever grateful to:

Jim Ciaravella, MD (retired pediatric cardio-thoracic surgeon) – for his incredible artistic talents in his creation of an original painting flawlessly depicting our title.

Susan Frederick – for her editing and undying encouragement to make this a reality. She has been a pillar of strength and positivity to us.

Devon Morgan of PhotoSynthesis Studio – for her preparation and adaptation of our artist's conception into the cover of our book.

Especially for that young family who journeyed to the seventh floor Ortho clinic (not once but twice) to carry the message that I am blessed to bring to each of you.

WHERE DO DOCTORS HIDE THEIR WINGS?

# CONTENTS

# INTRODUCTION

WHAT SEEMS NOW TO HAVE been many years ago, while working at the V.A. Hospital in St. Louis, I had the opportunity to share thoughts with a hospital Chaplin, Father Bill. He and I shared many discussions and I often called on him for his counsel and blessings for our men and women of the armed services and their families.

Among our personal discussions, he occasionally brought up my work schedule and the frequency with which we both found ourselves at a veteran's bedside. Among his comments was the speculation that physicians and related professionals would be better off celibate. I spontaneously rejected the thought (of course!) but later on began to appreciate Father Bill's remarks. Medicine, he explained, is not unlike the ministry. The expectations of those who seek our help are often disproportionate to our ability to fulfill them, and rarely can we do them justice without a great deal of sacrifice on the part of our families because of our already over-taxed time and attention.

At the time, I didn't realize how prophetic his remarks were and how I would come to recall them time and time again. By 2003, while working to create McKenna Project and *The Martial Art of Medicine* seminars, I shared with my team some of the stories and experiences that had punctuated my training. It was then that they said, "You really need to record those, and maybe even write a book!"

Decades had passed since I had begun my pursuit to become a healer, when late one Friday afternoon I found myself alone in an orthopedic clinic. This book was in draft in my mind but very much alive in my heart.

At the end of the day when only the clerical staff remained on the floor and I was awaiting my last patient, a young African American family came down the hall: A man of about twenty-eight, his wife and their relatively newborn son in his mother's arms.

We greeted one another and the man accompanied me to an exam room while his family stayed back in the adjacent waiting area – ostensibly so that mom could feed her son.

In the exam room I pursued his history, complaints or symptoms and I examined him before turning him over to the x-ray technologist for examination of his boney anatomy.

When he returned, we reviewed the films and my findings and recommendations to his satisfaction. When we stood to part, he interrupted me, "You're a writer, aren't you!," he blurted.

I was startled and paused long enough for him to repeat, "You are a writer – are you not?"

"Well", I replied, "I don't really know what to say about that, but I have been working on the idea of writing a book." My patient interrupted me, "Write the book," he said, and then he added, "I even know what the title should be!"

"Really?" I responded. "Yes, yes," he seemed even more excited, "You should call it: 'Where Do Doctors Hide Their Wings?'"

In disbelief and shock I promised I would and thanked him for his confidence and encouragement. We shook hands and left the room to join his family. In the waiting area my young friend announced 'our decision' and his wife enthusiastically agreed.

As they departed, I was overwhelmed with the whole experience and could not stop replaying the events in my mind the rest of the evening. Time passed and I began in seriousness to pen the first draft of my life's work. It took almost a year but I managed to record a rough version of the first 12 chapters and was determined to make it happen.

A year later to the month, I found myself in the same clinic one Friday afternoon and unbelievably the same scenario occurred. The same couple came down the hall with their now toddler in a stroller. I confess I didn't recognize them. Even the similarity of events evaded me until we sat down together in the exam room.

My patient looked at me and simply asked: "Did you write the book?" At that moment it all came back. "Yes," I replied, "at least the first draft in about a dozen chapters."

"Great," he added shaking my hand. "Now finish it and spread the word. 'Where Do Doctors Hide Their Wings?'" I interrupted him to ask about his knee injury. He happily reported it had returned to normal.

We talked with his wife and I met their son with hugs and handshakes. We parted after a very warm and cordial conversation. On the way out he said, "I won't be back again."

CHAPTER 1

# PIGEONS ON MY CHEST

I N ANOTHER TIME AND PLACE, forty years ago, I began
my foray into the world of medicine. In some ways it was
more primitive than medicine today, although oddly
enough, some things haven't changed at all since then. For
me, being a student in that world was an unforgettable experience. At times it seemed as if the journey would never end,
and at times I wondered if I could survive it. For most of my
twenty-four months in training, culminating in my graduation as a Physician Assistant, I lived in a single call room on
the third floor of Valley Hospital.

My colleagues knew the call room as "Dennis lives here,"
and apparently the name stuck, for so it remained during six
more years of P.A. hopefuls. It was more like a large closet
than a room, not more than twelve feet from threshold to
windowsill and about eight feet wide. There was a single, clear
light bulb hanging from a black wire that was attached to the
junction box twelve or fifteen feet off the floor. There was no
fan and no air conditioning in the call rooms, or the entire
hospital for that matter. We all kept our windows open, day
and night, rain or shine, winter or summer. The terrazzo slabs
that floored the entire building were heated with steam pipes.

It was so hot in summer that I assumed the heat was on year-round. I didn't know that for sure, of course, because I never allowed my unshod foot to touch the floor. I was aware that no mop (wet or dry) had ever touched it either.

Neither did I dare to shower in the co-ed bathroom, for fear of being happened upon by a member of the opposite sex. Actually, I think there were both Men's and Women's bathrooms, but the lack of security in the building permitted anyone to walk in twenty-four hours a day. In fact, it may have been that lack of security which prompted the fairer sex to use the Men's room, in hopes that one of their male colleagues would be there for protection, or come along relatively soon to dissuade interlopers.

The entire building was tiled with subway tile, much in vogue back then. It extended from the terrazzo floor to the nine-foot level and also above the doorways, which were in-set alcoves to allow the doors to open without restricting the traffic/stretchers/visitors and criminals who roamed the halls more night than day. The subway tile was a dingy mustard color. When coupled with the yellowed milk-glass globes that festooned the center of the ceiling every 100 feet, it gave the whole place a dark and creepy B-movie look.

I was jealous of my colleagues who spent most of their time in the comparative luxury of the Veterans Administration Hospitals in the "better" neighborhoods of St. Louis. But, despite the gloomy atmosphere of Valley Hospital, there was a camaraderie that developed among those of us assigned there. I got to know literally everyone in this incredibly massive institution. It was huge, an entire city block on every side

– North, South, East and West – four square blocks with a courtyard in the middle.

The courtyard was an unsightly mess with thirty years' clutter from patients, visitors and professional students who apparently chose to use the windows as refuse receptacles. As a result, the courtyard was littered with everything from used condoms to wine bottles and landscaped with a few (mostly dead) trees, shrubs, and various and sundry weeds. During my time there, at least four patients or visitors jumped from a window to their death in that courtyard. Fortunately, for all concerned, the maintenance staff (loosely entitled) always called the police to assist in a hasty removal of the corpse from the courtyard to the morgue, in the basement of our esteemed hospital. But it was clear that human debris was the only kind that warranted an immediate removal.

Sleep at Valley Hospital was rare, in always-brief snippets, and welcomed. At least the sheets were clean, although the room might have qualified as a hotel room in Hell, and hotter, I'm sure, than Satan himself would tolerate. That's why we never closed the windows. No one worried if it rained in. Rain was rare in St. Louis in the summer. And in winter – even though the weather was cold, icy and snowy – we still kept the windows cracked for a semblance of "fresh" air, such as it was. Not to say that the hospital had a bad aroma, but, a few blocks south, a brewery wafted its ever-present smell of cooking hops. Eventually we got to know the odor, but at first I couldn't determine what that "stink" was.

It was my fellow student and partner in crime, Hal, who informed me about the brewery landmark that was our most influential neighbor. Hal was a native of St. Louis, a Vietnam

Marine vet and the funniest madman I'd ever met. His method of coping with adverse circumstances was humor, along with a plethora of knowledge in the laboratory sciences. He had an edge on the rest of us since he'd worked in that department at Valley Hospital a few years earlier.

Hal was always injecting absurdities into the stresses of our experiences. He cajoled me once into rigging up a stretcher with a dummy we'd covered in sheets that trailed loosely on all four sides. We then convinced the hospital operator to page repeatedly, *"Doctor Howard, Doctor Fine, Doctor Howard"* as we raced through the halls of the hospital screaming the *"woo-woo-wahoo-woo"* chant made famous by the "Three Stooges" (probably too long ago for most of you to remember). Nevertheless, the act was a stunning success. As we rounded the turn into the wards, suddenly everyone – the nurses, residents and students writing up their patient histories, studying, or even dozing with their heads flat against the cold steel table (a smattering of drool leaking from their lips) – was wide awake and falling to the famed terrazzo floor, writhing with laughter! And laughter, like sleep, was a priceless commodity.

Hal was more than comic relief. He worked with conviction and gratitude for the opportunity to serve the sick rather than to have "bought it" in Vietnam. He was tireless in his clinical studies, and together we shared the seemingly endless task of admitting new patients each night, plus the routine of caring for those already on our unit. We made trip after trip to the lab to carry phlebotomy samples and plate cultures, and we ferried blood transfusions to the many people in dire need of supplementation for anemias, gunshot wounds, gastrointestinal bleeds and God-only-knows what else.

We traveled together for companionship and to lighten the burden when there was literally too much for one pair of arms to carry. When at last the work was done and quiet crept onto the floor, our Unit I Chief Resident, Joe, would demonically announce a 3 a.m. teaching session. Eventually, Joe would tire of the late night game and tell us to go on up to bed to get some sleep, but be back early enough to see patients before breakfast and do morning rounds at 8:00 a.m. As we tumbled into the clean sheets of our call rooms around 4:00 or 5:00 a.m., sleep was short and precious.

Our call rooms were on the third floor. Two small elevators that ran only during the daytime controlled access to that level. So, before we could crash, we had to hike up six flights of terrazzo stairs. The telephone operator was our only alarm clock and gave accommodating wake-up calls at 6:30 a.m., and again at 6:45. It felt odd to sleep alone, away from my wife of less than two years, but then again, I wasn't actually alone. Because of the always-open window, I often awakened to intimate company – pigeons –usually two or three watching me from the iron rail at the foot of my bed, another perched on the windowsill, and almost always one on my chest.

If the University had known, I would have probably been dropped from the program for having pets.

CHAPTER 2

# STERILIZED FLYSWATTERS

E ARLY ON IN MY EXPERIENCES at Valley Hospital, I became acquainted with the dangers of the open door policy of this hospital. It was so large that all the medical school professors had offices and research labs on the fourth floor in the back of the hospital, and a kennel and dog lab existed on the roof. While on Unit II Surgery, I got to know and work under Dr. Ed. Dr. Ed was a hard-nosed Vietnam trained trauma surgeon who drove a mid-engine Porsche and carried a .357 magnum in the glove box. He supported his chief resident and the rest of us the way a master sergeant looks after his troops.

No matter what the hour, if we needed him, he was out of bed and on his way to the hospital. Lacking the sophisticated scans and angiograms we have today, the chief resident frequently found himself faced with dilemmas only Dr. Ed could solve. And solve them he did, many times, in the wee hours between dark and dawn. Once we raced a patient who was clearly bleeding to death to the operating room, yet he did not have a scratch on him. Once on the table, Dr. Ed rushed into the room asking questions in rapid-fire haste in order to solve the conundrum and save the patient. When no solution was obvious, he ordered us to turn the patient on his belly and shoved a gloved hand up the man's rectum to return a fistful of clots. "They shot him up his rectum," he shouted. "Turn him back over and open him from xyphoid to pubis."

We did, and it worked! I was in awe. But in the medical world, awe is quickly tempered with a strong dose of reality. My dose that night was the privilege of learning, hands-on, as Dr. Will, the chief resident, stood by patiently, how to anastamose each of the bowel resections we had been forced to perform.

It wasn't much more than a week later that another citizen was wheeled in: the critical victim of a drug deal gone bad. Dr. Will was already in the emergency room treating one of the patient's colleagues. Dr. Ed had driven to the hospital to get the first case started. As long as I live I will not forget what happened that night. It was 4:00 a.m. and Dr. Ed and I scrubbed up while we watched the O.R. nurses set up the instruments and the anesthesiologist prepare to "sleep the patient," who was already stripped naked, belted to the table and smeared copiously with antiseptic.

It was surrealistically silent for a moment. Suddenly, we were both aware of the sound of metal elevator doors opening in the corridor directly across the way. I remember wondering if Dr. Will was coming up from the E.R., but in a blinding flash I felt Dr. Ed's large, wet hand slap the back of my neck. I crumpled to the terrazzo floor as he screamed, "DOWN, DOWN, EVERYBODY DOWN!"

The next thing I heard was ear piercing. Two shotguns went off in rapid succession, casings clanking to the floor. Seconds later the elevator doors closed and silence returned.

When I got to my feet, what had formerly been a human torso had been ripped and torn by shotgun blasts until only the belted portion remained. Still stunned, I asked Dr. Ed how he knew what was about to happen. He explained that no one would be on that elevator at this hour without sinister business in mind. And, in situations like this, it was not uncommon for assailants to come in to "finish the job."

Many days, and even more nights, were spent in the operating room with my mentors and friends, learning about life and medicine. The operating room became a sort of sanctuary for me. I discovered a perennial jar of peanut butter and saltines that stayed in the storage room between the O.R.'s where I could get a snack in the middle of the night, between patients or just before the long trek to my call room for a short sleep.

The absence of air conditioning and screens on the windows presented us with a recurring irony in the operating room. The open window served as an irresistible temptation to countless flies, no doubt attracted by the waft of cooking hops at the nearby brewery.

Predictably then, while we were surgically examining, say, the entrails of some hapless patient, a fly (or flies) would threaten our sterile field. For our defense, the nurses had decided unilaterally to prepare an ample supply of flyswatters, fully sterilized and packed alongside the instruments, for just such occasions. I was used to the surgeon's barking commands as he requested instruments he needed, but it took everything I had not to hit the terrazzo surface once again in uncontrollable laughter when I heard him yell "Flyswatter!"

CHAPTER 3

# POCKET ON FIRE

D IVISION II MEDICINE WAS IN no way similar to my previous experience. In fact, I took the assignment as a kind of insult stemming from an unexplainable dislike of me by the P.A. Program Director. One day, secreted away in an empty classroom, I confidentially confessed my complaints to Doug, commonly perceived as the students' best friend.

Doug had been a student in the very first P.A. class, his graduation delayed by an auto accident that bought him a fractured femur and a job as Assistant Director in the interim.

Although he finished the program in year two with the second class, he was retained as Assistant Director and loved by all.

Doug listened kindly to my disgruntlement, promising confidentiality. But within an hour I was summoned to the office of the Chief of Unit II Medicine. Dr. Gert was from Germany. He wore wire rimmed glasses and smoked incessantly, a cigarette pinched between his thumb and forefinger in a backhanded fashion.

Petrified at being called to his inner sanctum, I sat numbly in the antiquated wooden chair he pointed me to across from his desk. Speaking loudly in his thick German accent, he roared, "Soooo, you don't like it here, do you?"

My protests were smothered by his "Velll, ve shall seeee!" He tossed a piece of paper at me across the top of his desk. On it was scribbled, "180-90-120-130-70-11." He looked at me and demanded, "Vaaat is dis?" I didn't have a clue. "DIABEETEEES!" he roared.

"Now!" he ordered, "Vee vill teach you medicine so you vill not feel cheated, yah? You vill meet here vith me on Vednesday, und next door vith Dr. Rama on Thursdays from 1600-1700 hours every veek for the next sixteen veeks, yah?" With this, I stood up in a spontaneous version of military attention. "Yes, sir. Thank you, sir," I said, and quickly exited in a full sweat.

The following rotation was painful, but incredibly valuable. My two mentors seemed to take on my medical education as a personal challenge and were bent on my absorbing everything they knew. They even tried to outdo one another in the process. The hourly sessions often became an hour and a half or two, after which I had to hurry back to the wards to finish my day's work, encountering one or the other of them again on evening rounds.

Dr. Gert still smoked everywhere in the hospital, even at the bedside of patients while he was doing teaching rounds. If the ash on his cigarette got too long, it would fall off onto the patient's sheet-draped belly. On one occasion he flicked the ash into the pocket of his white professorial lab coat, where it soon began to smolder. Dr. Gert paid no attention. He was talking, teaching and gesticulating to us as the smoke grew stronger and stronger. Our student eyes were all riveted on the impending disaster, as were the patient's. Finally,

I grabbed a cup of water from the patient's night stand and doused the now somewhat blackened pocket. My impetuous action brought a moment of terror to my colleagues, but Dr. Gert only gave me a cold stare and continued with his lecture.

Tension and lighthearted hilarity often traded places as we went through our days. At that time it was still widely held that pneumococcal pneumonia was a virulent disease and, in order to treat it successfully, early diagnosis and antibiotics were necessary. The laboratory methods using culture sensitivity were fairly slow so an older method was still employed on Unit II.

Dr. Gert had taught me that in medicine you must unlearn two things that your mother taught you never to do: Stare and Ask Questions! That is how I discovered the faster method of diagnosing pneumococcal. Another German doctor, a resident, was happy to explain it to me. "Vhen you admit a patient with suspected pneumonia, it is important to determine vhether it is pneumococcal or not. Soooo, you draw the blood from the patient and inject it into a mouse. If it is pneumococcus the mouse will be dead in 12 hours." (Each division of the hospital had a small lab that provided the opportunity to plate cultures, spin hematocrits, examine blood smears, and do rudimentary urinalyses. In addition to these was a small cage next to the window, refreshed daily with small white mice.)

I saw this "mouse method" in action about three weeks later. Among our troop was a Greek resident who was pleasant enough, but with whom I had not had much contact. He had apparently admitted a patient with pneumonia and drawn blood to inject into the hind quarters of an unsuspecting (and very cute) little white mouse (with red eyes). Although I didn't witness the actual injection, I suddenly heard a blood curdling scream. The 6' 6" Greek doctor, dressed from head to toe in whites, was bolting through the open doorway with a little white mouse dangling from his hand, teeth firmly imbedded in the web between thumb and forefinger. The little guy had obviously retaliated!

Laughter erupted in the room – no, it was beyond laughter! Students were actually falling on the floor grasping their mid-sections in hilarity at the sight of this huge man at the mercy of his tiny victim.

Having a secret affinity for all kinds of animals (it started in the second grade when my teacher read a chapter of Dr. Doolittle to us every afternoon), the idea of subjecting a defenseless creature to the pain of injection and possible death just to save a few hours didn't seem like a worthy tradeoff. I opted to give the antibiotics to the patient and the cultures to the lab.

## CHAPTER 4

# 27 SHOCK TREATMENTS

I N RETROSPECT, IT SEEMS THAT my experiences represented a panoply of challenges, some sad and sorrowful, some joyfully successful, but sprinkled with frightening and almost slapstick comedic events. Maybe fatigue played a bigger role than I remembered, but the intensity of each episode was permanently seared into my soul.

One such cascade of events began one weekend on Division II Medicine. Dr. Hans and I were on call that Saturday night and we had had a particularly busy day. We also inherited a number of patients from departing staff members who had hurriedly signed out their patients to us and rushed off to savor a rare evening at home. Among them was a man whose plight was alcoholism-related cirrhosis of the liver. That was all that our Greek friend (the mouse-killer) had relayed in the process of turning over his thirty-some patients to us for his share of our night's work.

The first thing to do when assuming care of some seventy patients for the night is to try to assess their condition and the immediate needs they might have in the hours to come. That alone took hours, as our little team of two briefly examined each patient and their charts. In the process we encountered the patient with cirrhosis, whose jaundiced skin, yellow eyes and protuberant belly displayed his serious condition. He did not respond to our attempts to communicate with him.

With that noted, we moved on and a couple of hours later reviewed our notes and plans for the evening. First up was the blood-letting with seemingly endless tubes, labels, plastic bags and completed request forms that I, naturally, was expected to take to the lab. We went about seeing and admitting new patients from the emergency room. It was near midnight before the results had arrived at the nursing station for us to sort through and affix to each patient's chart.

Coming upon our newly acquired yellow man's numbers, we were shocked to find a dangerously elevated potassium level of 7.0 and a similarly high creatinine level. It was clear that his liver failure had reached a crisis point as a result of fluid loss into the abdomen. That information was, at that point in our careers, about all we knew about late-stage liver disease. Dr. Hans got out his Washington University Medical Manual, however, and we promptly poured over it in search of answers to the impending crisis. We first suspected an error in the life-threatening potassium elevation, but the Wash U. manual suggested a 12-lead EKG to confirm the finding in an instantly available modality. We did one. To our surprise the tracing was an exact copy of the one depicted in the text. An ominous spread-out wavy line extended from left to right.

Quickly we referred to the venerated manual, which recounted the practice of giving kayexcelate enemas to lower the patient's potassium level. We administered these enemas personally throughout the remainder to the night, to no avail. We had tried and failed. He died there in a bed littered with stool coated towels, surrounded by on-lookers who sat in silence on the edges of their beds, staring at the curtained drama within as the two of us pleaded with the Universe for assistance. Beaten, feeling defeated and truly exhausted, we left our patient for the staff to transport to the morgue, and headed for bed.

Two hours later I was awakened by the nurse from the Unit. "You'd better get down here right away," she blurted. I jumped to my feet, fearing another catastrophe had befallen us. As I arrived on the unit I was immediately confronted by the image of Dr. Gert sitting at the stainless steel table and backhanding a cigarette to his lips. "Can I get you anything?" I asked. "Caaffeee," he replied, and then he repeated his oft-quoted expression, "Black as an Ethiopian, Sweet as..." (I asked him once where he got the quote and he told me it was from Omar Khayyam. Since then, I have yet to find the quote or remember the rest of the expression he used, but nonetheless it was vintage Dr. Gert.)

Alerted to the night nurse's recount of the previous night's events, he immediately announced that we would discuss that later, and began rounds in that predawn Sunday morning.

Finishing at about 10:00 a.m., Dr. Gert took Dr. Hans and me aside, announcing that he would like to take us to breakfast in Clayton, Missouri – a nearby suburb of St. Louis – and we gratefully and reluctantly accepted.

I remember calling my wife to alert her that I would be home late. Normally we attended church together on Sunday morning, an event I especially relied on for spiritual sustenance during those days. It always gave us a sense of "centering," and I interpreted the weekly collection basket as a sort of omen. Each Sunday, when the basket came around, I would reach into my pocket and produce a dollar bill. It was always my last and only dollar bill, but somehow on Monday a few more would turn up.

My wife was gracious and encouraged my attendance at brunch so Dr. Hans and I cautiously climbed into Dr. Gert's Porsche. The silence was thick as we motored away from the steps of Valley Hospital. Shortly thereafter he broke the moment with, "Sooo... vhat happened?"

Dr. Hans recounted the events, and I interjected a minimum of affirmations to support him. Dr. Gert asked me directly if Dr. Hans had accurately depicted the happenings of the night. I reiterated that he had.

Arriving at the restaurant, we climbed out of the car and went inside to sit down to brunch with continued apprehension, but the conversation never returned to the patient and his demise. Instead, for the next three hours, Dr. Gert lectured us on the diagnosis and management of hyperkalemia in patients with end-stage cirrhosis with hepato-renal syndrome. We listened intently, ate a great brunch appreciatively, and learned the secrets of success in the circumstances we had just encountered. To this very day it is carved into my soul that had we given IV glucose and IV insulin in rapid succession, we would probably have gotten the potassium down precipitously. The patient would have likely died at a later date, however, from the same thing or another complication of his disease.

During this era of my training, I spent most of my time alone. I missed the support and company of Hal and my other classmates, and that sense of separation from my group loomed over me heavily. But, in retrospect, it was all for the best since Dr. Gert and Dr. Rama gave me private tutoring every afternoon. I was also forced to work more closely with the residents on my teams.

Even so, the experiences of previous times with Hal and friends continued to contribute to my life. One of those was a fellow Hal had introduced to me who ran the blood bank there at Valley Hospital. They called him "House" for reasons that were immediately obvious. Indeed, he was as big as a house and frighteningly dour and sinister in appearance. I discovered that House had once been a patient of the hospital, in fact, not just once. He had, on many different occasions, been a frequent guest of the psychiatric ward, which was housed in a building across the street from our emergency room and was equally ominous in appearance. I had once had the misfortune of going there alone for a medical consult. It was because of that experience that I could never bring myself to view the movie, *One Flew Over the Cuckoo's Nest*, some years later. Even the previews were all too familiar.

House had been hospitalized for paranoid schizophrenia numerous times and received 27 ECT's – electroconvulsive treatments – commonly known as shock treatments. I knew that even a singular ECT experience could impact one's animation and personality, but knowing House, I became convinced that the results of many treatments are decidedly cumulative.

A low groan was House's response to almost any salutation. He rarely made eye contact. His face was entirely expressionless. It never wrinkled with laughter or smiles. Hal had known him for years and my association with Hal must have given me a measure of acceptance with him when we were first introduced. Later, on Unit II Medicine, my visits to the blood bank became solo, and in my isolation I found a sort of sanctuary there with House. I took a few minutes each time to have a cigarette and a cup of coffee with him. We didn't need to talk. In fact, the silence was precious. It's interesting what comrades we find when we are lonely, and how indelibly comforting those few moments with another lonely human being can become.

CHAPTER 5

# AN ARMFUL OF HARD EARNED BLOOD

YOU MIGHT THINK IT A simple task to master the skill of phlebotomy (blood drawing), especially since my daily routine included drawing endless samples from those least likely to have drug-free backgrounds, resulting in copious large veins, which by all counts should have been easy to "hit." Sadly, this was not the case. Vein puncture in that setting was laborious, embarrassing and often next to impossible. The heat alone – real or imagined – caused streams of perspiration to run down my face and the patients could feel my anxiety making the task all the more difficult.

Regardless, it was a challenge I was forced to come to grips with day-in and day-out. The tension was heightened by nurses, who, out of a sense of protecting their patients, liked to announce as I struggled to pierce the cephalic vein, "You only get three chances!"

On one such occasion, I had garnered an armload of blood samples at the early hour of 2:00 a.m. and started my lonely trek down the center hall toward the laboratory and my private sanctuary: the blood bank. The hall was dark and empty. Each doorway alcove was a potential hazard so I carried my valuable cargo with authority (and a great deal of caution) past the darkened alcoves.

As I neared the left turn at the end of the hall, feeling relieved to have passed the last doorway, a man suddenly appeared from the right side of the corridor which led to the emergency room. As he walked toward me, I noticed his reluctance to look at me, a silent signal I perceived as threatening.

With both my arms loaded with lab samples, I was about to pass him when he turned to grab me. I remember his jacket, a maroon high school letter jacket sans insignias, with cream-colored leather sleeves. I caught those sleeves as I threw all the samples at his face and swung him around with all my weight, slamming his shoulder against the mustard-colored subway tile behind me.

The side of his head struck the tile wall making a resounding pumpkin-like thump. Immediately, he went limp, slumping to the floor. I rounded the corner and took off for the lab at a dead run.

Inside the blood bank, I locked the door behind me and fell into a chair across from the lab table where House sat, blank faced, as always.

He stared at me and waited. Once I'd caught my breath and gotten some blood back into my brain, I was able to tell him what had happened. He said nothing, just picked up the phone to call the E.R. He talked to the "Turn Key," one of three city police officers stationed in the E.R. to keep the peace and, when necessary, lock up any boisterous citizens until the paddy wagon could come to cart them away.

House greeted the cop dryly and informed him that some character had tried to "rough up one of my friends," and could be found unconscious or dead in the main corridor. He hung up the phone, brought me a cup of coffee, gave me one of his cigarettes and eventually walked me back to the floor by a different route through the basement.

After my coffee and cigarette recovery, I returned to the business of re-drawing all those blood samples.

I never heard another word about the guy who had attacked me that night.

CHAPTER 6

# BOTTLE O' WINE

I T'S HARD TO OVERSTATE THE influence that Dr. Gert had upon me. His scientific knowledge and theories – as well as practical approaches – were amazingly effective. I recall his lecture at the bedside of a patient who had suffered a heart attack, a myocardial infarction. It is now referred to as a "silent M.I." or a "non-Q wave M.I." (one that doesn't show up on the EKG). Dr. Gert stated that he would someday like to set up a series of experiments to treat myocardial infarctions with an aspirin I.V. He was always discussing the etiology or pathophysiology of such events as "white thrombi" or "platelet thrombi."

Remember, all this occurred in 1973. Today it is a standard procedure when admitting a patient with chest pain – in order to rule out myocardial infarction – to have the patient chew an aspirin in the emergency room. The sublingual veins in the mouth are known to transport nitroglycerine to the blood stream and subsequently the heart, also transporting acetylsalicylic acid to the heart, which may dissolve the platelet thrombus. Dr. Gert was one of those doctors who simply knew things ahead of time, before most other people knew them.

I remember one early morning during rounds when he came upon a patient that Dr. Hans and I were treating. Noting the history of alcoholism, and teaching us the pathophysiology that results from excessive alcohol use, he advised Librium, I.V. fluids with vitamins and I.M. injections of Thiamine 100 mg/day for the first three days, and by mouth thereafter.

By evening rounds the patient had worsened. Drenched with sweat, his pulse was 140 and he was picking at non-existent bugs on the bedclothes and shaking like a leaf in a tornado. Dr. Gert stood by the bedside and pointed out each of the symptoms, then ordered more Librium I.M.

Hours later, after Dr. Gert had been in his office for the evening, he returned and invited me to join him at the man's beside. He pointed out an increase in the pulse, more hallucinosis and behavior that had by this time bought him four-point leather restraints. Dr. Gert looked me in the eye and said, "This man may die. There is only one thing to do."

He reached into his pocket and produced a $5.00 bill. He handed it to me and said, "Go across the street and get a cheap bottle of wine and bring it back to me." Following his instructions, I ran a broken field pattern across the street into and out of the dingy little liquor store in front of the hospital.

Back on the Unit, Professor Gert sat at his favorite spot, drinking black coffee and smoking. He stood to collect his change, which he counted openly, and then took the bottle of wine to the patient's beside. He unscrewed the cap and handed the elixir to the grateful man, who survived to leave the hospital two days later in remarkably good shape.

<br>

CHAPTER 7

# ST. ELSEWHERE

A
FTER I SURVIVED THE RIGORS of three rotations at
Valley Hospital and two tours on Medicine I and II
– as well as a sixteen-week round of alternate night
call on Surgery Division II – I was finally assigned to Valley
Hospital for Children. This meant daytime and evening rotation without night call or sleeping in the hospital. For the first
time I looked forward to going home each night and seeing
my wife instead of merely catching up with her by phone at
odd hours.

The atmosphere at Valley Kids was different from Valley
Hospital. Everyone was more intense and not particularly
cordial or fun-loving. With a building full of little children
facing varying degrees of disease and all-too-frequently horrible outcomes, you can't expect a party. Pediatrics has a sad
side that is the most prominent aspect of a tertiary hospital like this one, and everyone in the building spends most
of their days trying to protect the children from anything or
anyone who would harm them.

There is a pervasive alertness for child abuse. That atmosphere greets you at the door. It is hammered into students to
look for *this* type of injury and *that* type of burn that typify

actual abuse, not accidents. There are lectures about pediatrics as a science, that is, not simply medicine applied to little people, but a unique arena with its own set of pitfalls to watch out for in the evaluation and treatment of children.

It's true. And while I was deeply impressed with the difference, I anticipated learning everything I could about the practice of medicine in pediatrics. Each morning, the Chairman of the Department of Radiology went over films at 6:00 a.m., and I was jammed into his tiny reading room every day to watch and listen. Every afternoon at 4:30 p.m. we met with Dr. Jim, the Chairman of the Department of Medicine. "Grand Rounds" was a daily affair for all medical residents, medical students and physician assistant students who filled the conference room from wall-to-wall.

Dr. Jim was a spellbinding teacher whose sincerity permeated the packed conference room. He sat at the head of a 30-foot table surrounded by chairs in which his residents, chief residents and staff members sat. Behind the chairs were the rest of us – medical students and physician assistant students – shoulder to shoulder, two and three deep, sitting on the familiar terrazzo floor.

Dr. Jim insisted on strict professionalism as each resident presented the admissions they had brought into the hospital during the past twenty-four hours. They were reminded often to refer to any outside institutions as "St. Elsewhere," so as not to impugn the integrity of another hospital or a private doctor's judgment.

The exercise allowed Dr. Jim to point out the diagnostic and examination skills required to determine treatment of each case. He emphasized that we must be vigilant never to admit a child to the hospital with chickenpox, as there were so many leukemics and immuno-suppressed patients for whom a case of chickenpox could be fatal.

Since child abuse management (termed CAM on posters throughout the hospital) was a frequent topic of conversation at Valley Kids, Dr. Jim was no stranger to its horrors. And he never missed an opportunity to point out the subtle nuances of clinical presentation, as well as the tragedy of overlooking them.

## CHAPTER 8

# BIG MISTAKE!

O N ONE PARTICULAR NIGHT (THESE late night brief-
ings were so thorough that they often went past
midnight), Dr. Jim asked our indulgence for a recount of a tragedy that one of his own residents had experienced. While working in the emergency room, this particular
resident was going from one exam area to another and was
surprised to find his own daughter on the exam table. He and
his wife were both medical residents and their nanny had
brought their infant daughter to the hospital with a broken
arm, specifically a broken humerus (the single, large bone in
the upper arm).

The resident confided to Dr. Jim that he had not suspected
anything, and splinting his daughter's arm, he sent her home
with the nanny. Everything appeared to be normal during
the recovery, and the child did well until another night weeks
later. Once again, he was staffing the emergency room when
an ambulance brought in a child whom he was pressed into
evaluating urgently. He entered the trauma exam room to
find his own little girl, dead.

All of us sat in stunned silence at an outcome too horrible to contemplate. I don't think anyone even breathed for a minute or two.

Dr. Jim took the time to review the details and the subtle hints that should have been apparent to the doctor when he saw his daughter the first time. He recounted the opportunities the resident had missed to identify child abuse in his own home, and he relayed to us the excruciating pain he felt for this couple as he attended their daughter's funeral.

It was a tragedy. And it hadn't happened at St. Elsewhere.

Somehow, that made it worse.

## CHAPTER 9

# ON THE TERRAZZO FLOOR

I T'S A DEEP EMPATHY ONE acquires simply from the everyday experiences in this setting. Everyone is somber, and rightly so. Each little helpless patient is totally dependent and trusting us, as medical people, to do the right thing. What makes us even more somber is that their parents feel equally helpless. They too, look to the hospital every day to take away their fears and insecurities about their little children.

Valley Kids never turned away a child who needed help. Everyone who brought a child to us was welcomed. No one ever questioned if the bill would be paid. In a midtown location, just blocks from the inner city, this little hospital was a giant in childcare. Mothers who were separated from the fathers of their children (often by Aid to Dependent Children regulations) got off the bus each night, brought dinner home to their children and then came to Valley Kids with one of the little ones who had become sick that day.

They waited by the dozens in what we called E.R. #2. This was a "sick kids" clinic that started at 2:00 p.m. and went to midnight or 1:00 a.m., or until all the children were seen. That was where I could be found every night throughout my stay at Valley Kids. We took histories from the moms, did physical exams on the children, presented the cases to a resident and, if he or she agreed, ordered x-rays or urinalyses or whatever seemed necessary. We prescribed medicine and/or admitted the child for further tests and treatment.

It was a process that required lots of communication between staff and mothers. The upshot was some serious development in the areas of empathy and respect for patients and parents, as well as endless second guessing of our own assessments so as not to let any of them down.

As the months went by, I traversed all the specialties. With every case I became more aware of what painful things can happen to children. I was deeply moved by all the people I encountered – Moms, Dads, Grandmas, and Grandpas – who hovered in the halls of the hospital and slept on the steam-heated terrazzo floors night after night, keeping the vigil, standing guard over their little ones.

The somber dignity and love evident here was quite a contrast to my previous experiences at Valley. Somehow I felt a kinship with these families. Something inside told me we shared something very basic, very human.

Little did I know that years later that feeling would return when my wife and I brought our little girl to a hospital some sixty miles east of St. Louis. She was lying in a croup tent with a 104 degree fever and signs of aseptic meningitis. We rushed her by ambulance from our local hospital to Valley Kids in St. Louis in the middle of the night, and the same Chief Resident I had studied under met us in the E.R. to admit her.

That night we joined the other parents on the warm and unyielding terrazzo floor – keeping vigil, not sleeping and praying for our daughter. The combination of our Chief Resident's

Herculean efforts coupled with our heartfelt prayers resolved our daughter's crisis readily and we returned home three days later.

CHAPTER 10

# SIXTY-DOLLARS-A-MINUTE STOPWATCH CHARLIE

TIME SLIPPED BY QUICKLY AS we traversed through graduation, board exams and the usual anti-climax of job search and the realities of professional life. It wasn't easy finding a position for a Physician Assistant in those early days. Many states had not enacted pertinent legislation and few physicians were willing to entertain the thought of hiring one, so it was an uphill climb.

We were still living with my wife's parents. I tumbled around Southern Illinois until I was finally interviewed and retained by a chap in the southeastern portion of the state. It was a nice location with a well-trained family practitioner named Charlie and a town that was friendly, although not replete with housing options.

One of the women in our office persuaded her husband to offer me their party trailer east of town on a forty-acre piece of land with a small lake, a barn and a fence. The accommodations were pleasant and cozy, at least until winter rolled in. I was there only at night and my wife stayed with her Mom and Dad while I scouted out the territory, looking for a proper place for us to rent. On weekends, I drove the thirty miles west to spend a couple of days with her and then return – always after dark – on Sunday nights.

After work each day, I snooped around town in search of likely places for us to live. Then, after eating at some local spot, I drove the many miles out to my tiny trailer in the dark. The nights were lonely and long so I always got up early to get to the office, do my rounds and grab a bite to eat before the day began.

One morning, after a particularly cold night and a furnace that was less than adequate, I got up even earlier than usual. I showered, shaved, dressed and stepped out the door onto the small wooden porch, which I noticed had turned to solid ice. I fumbled with the key to lock the trailer door behind me and stepped gingerly down the slippery stairs. I was reaching for the railing to steady myself when suddenly I was face to face with a huge animal. I screamed and tried hard to focus my eyes in the non-light of early morning. What I saw was the silhouette of a large, somewhat innocent horse-face reared back as though equally terrified. Apparently, Mr. and Mrs. D. had failed to inform me that I was not alone out there in the middle of nowhere – and, having never seen the place in the daylight – I had not suspected that I shared the property with anyone, human or otherwise. Later that morning when I relayed my surprised terror to the doctor and his office staff, they were in stitches with laughter. Only at that point was I alerted by my hostess that I had equine companions that lived with me on the property – not just one, but TWO of them.

Eventually, we found a place to rent and moved into town to become a part of the community. Charlie, the doctor, was a good guy. His practice, his wife and the community seemed great, and we were very busy, working shoulder-to-shoulder, stamping out disease.

After awhile, I began to discern more about how the practice worked and was amazed to see a heavy emphasis on payment for services. Patients with an outstanding balance were very fairly, but in a business-like fashion, turned over to small claims court as soon as it was apparent they were not paying in a timely fashion. A few months after I had settled into my new routine, Doctor Charlie suggested that I consider adopting the rather innovative billing method that he had developed.

He explained that that there was a gadget with five plastic arms folded against the doorframe that he extended in a color-coded pattern when he went into an examining room. This indicated he was with the patient. As he entered the room, he would zero out a stopwatch he carried on a shoelace, click it to start and hang it over the extended plastic indicators.

When he emerged from the room, he would check the stopwatch and charge according to the time elapsed. In this manner, he never felt the need to rush a patient. Instead, he allowed them to talk on and on, as long as they wished. He simply charged them for every minute. (My wife reminded me recently that the charge was $60 a minute.) With this system, patients who got right to the point and did not dally paid less than those who did. I confess I was a bit taken aback by his system, but it worked well for him and I never heard a patient grumble. They gladly paid for every minute he listened and when they did not, they went to court.

## CHAPTER 11

# DON'T WORRY – IF YOU'RE ARRESTED, WE'LL SUE 'EM

I NEVER DID ADOPT THE STOPWATCH method, but my practice flourished on a flat rate charge that we both determined was fair. My wife and I had ready access to her family and we were rapidly absorbed into our new community. Life was good!

It wasn't long before my wife became pregnant. But very early on she began spotting with an ischemic-threatened miscarriage and wound up spending every day, all day, on the couch in the apartment.

Work for me was fine, but not too significant in our order of priorities as a couple. Days were pretty routine. Then one evening I received a call from my boss. He informed me that he was going out of town to a meeting and asked me to keep the office going in his absence, as well as check on the patients in the hospital. As he was about to hang up he remarked, almost as an aside, "Oh, and if they come to arrest you for criminal trespassing, go quietly. We'll sue 'em later."

I got off the phone, looked at my couch-ridden wife, and wondered out loud what that last comment might mean.

She suggested I call him right back to clarify precisely what he meant.

That's exactly what I did. Minutes later I was standing at his back door waiting to talk the whole thing over so I could gain an accurate appreciation of his proposal and make my first big decision as a husband and potential father. We sat in his family room drinking his scotch and arguing into the wee small hours over our dilemma. Unbeknownst to me, Charlie and his colleagues at the hospital had been waging war for months over my presence in the community. They debated its effect upon their own practices and the advisability of this new profession called "physician assistants" when the state had yet to recognize them legally.

The debate had reached such a heated point that they declared they would have me arrested the next time I saw a patient in the hospital! It was at this point that Charlie decided he had better fill me in. The more he described the situation, the more incensed I became. The implications were devastating, not only for my little family, but for my entire profession.

It was difficult, but despite the scotches, I was clear-headed. I informed him I would be looking elsewhere for employment immediately. He argued and offered to defend me to the other physicians in the community, but I would hear nothing of it. Clearly, he had brought me into a situation that was hazardous for me and my family without letting me know in advance of the potential dangers. For me it was a simple matter of broken trust. I felt betrayed. There was no going back.

The next day I went to see the hospital administrator to tell him what had happened the night before. He apologized, but I insisted he inform the other medical staff that I had no desire to go to jail for anyone, and that I would not step foot in the hospital again. This defused the situation. With the return of my boss from his trip, I resumed seeing patients only in his presence in the office and began my search for alternatives. My boss, I must say, was remorseful in regard to what had happened and appeared not to blame me for my stubbornness. Whenever I had an opportunity, he gladly gave me an excellent reference and was a real gentleman about my leaving.

## CHAPTER 12

# DIAGNOSTIC PALM READING

I N FAIRLY SHORT ORDER WE got resettled in another
community and another family practice setting. My ev-
er-so-pregnant wife and I moved into a nice little two-bed-
room house we rented only a few blocks from our new office. I
felt comfortable working for a man who had a recent academ-
ic background at the University of Illinois Medical School,
and I was also determined to work for the establishment of
legislation in Illinois that would stabilize my profession.

I volunteered to serve on the legislative committee for
the Illinois Academy of Physician Assistants and drove to
Springfield every Wednesday to roam the halls of the statehouse, shaking hands and introducing myself to everyone
who would stand still long enough. Eventually, our committee
met up with the lobbyist for the Illinois State Medical Society.
He quite literally helped us draft the necessary legislation and
taught us how to introduce it for a vote.

We worked together for months while my good wife was
at home growing our daughter and decorating a nursery. We
were busy and happy and going along in a civilized manner.
Summer turned to fall, and somewhere during the change
of seasons my boss's partner unexpectedly resigned! He told

the boss he wanted to go out West to be a cowboy and a doctor both. Looking back, we should have had a clue. The guy always dressed like a cowboy, right down to his matching pearl-handled .45 caliber six shooters that he wore on weekends at festivals. So the wanna-be cowboy doctor left and things got busier for the doc and myself.

About that time, my friend – the lobbyist – called me to the State Legislature. When I arrived, I encountered him on the statehouse floor. The room was deserted except for the two of us. He sadly informed me that the previous night he had met with the ISMS and been directed to block the passage of our bill. He explained the trepidation some less-confident physicians had expressed about competing with P.A.s. I, of course, protested loudly and with some emotion, "What nonsense!"

"Calm down, calm down," he chided. "You and I are just going to go have lunch while the legislature is in session. And, hey, whatever happens while we're gone, happens."

Although I was anxious over the developments in the office back home, the impending delivery of our daughter and this threat to scuttle our last eight months of legislative preparation, I decided I was willing to trust my new friend. So we had lunch, and while we ate, the legislature passed the Physician Assistant Bill. My profession gained official recognition in the state of Illinois due to the well-intentioned (and strategically designed) neglect of a good guy.

Over the next few weeks, things began to get strange at the office. The boss wanted to sue the partner for leaving. I encouraged him to be gracious despite the inconvenience his leaving caused us. The delivery of our daughter was nearing and I took my wife to her mother's to be near her doctor for the event. I would drive the 150 miles to be there with her myself when the time came. In between false alarms and hurried drives (only to turn back on Sunday evening), my boss decided to make use of the office his former partner had vacated. He entered into an agreement with a palm reader, a woman who claimed to be able to read a woman's palm print and tell if she already had breast cancer, ever will have breast cancer or never will have breast cancer.

This piece of news was so disturbing that, although my wife was due to deliver any day, I could not escape a conversation with the boss about his new employee. He informed me calmly that it was none of my business, and that he was doing it as an experiment. When a patient came in to see him regarding a lump in her breast, he examined her first and then had her meet the palm reader, who made a print of the palm for the chart and give her impression of the diagnosis.

I deferred to his judgment and busied myself with the birth of our new daughter and her christening. It was early March when I spoke with my boss again. This time I was more direct and stated my candid feeling that palm reading was unprofessional, medically speaking, and therefore unfair to our patients. He disagreed with my input. In a few short weeks we were packing our things – again.

CHAPTER 13

# THE SAWED-OFF SHOTGUN NEIGHBOR

I WAS IN A QUANDARY AS to what direction to take. As I reviewed my options, I felt compelled to take a few days to go back to my hometown of Chicago and see what prospects that might hold.

We took our little daughter and visited my parents in Chicago for two weeks as I tapped the city, interviewing with anyone who would listen to me. At the end of the two weeks I had no new prospects, no job, no place to live and a brand new daughter now four months old.

Returning home to boxes of things half-packed, I continued to mentally strategize about my next move. We were out in the yard gathering up things from the garage one afternoon, and our neighbor came by to ask, "What's this? Are you packing up?" I didn't answer immediately because I was distracted by the very big gun he was swinging back and forth in his right hand. "What the hell is that?" I asked. "A mean-shooter," he replied, "I always carry this when I'm out driving truck." Turning to go, he shot back a "Good luck" over his shoulder and I went into the house to pack our belongings with renewed fervor.

WHERE DO DOCTORS HIDE THEIR WINGS?

No matter how disappointed I had been in our first two jobs out of school – and no matter how much I felt it had been my fault that each in turn had been a disaster – there clearly was no good reason to wish that we could stay.

On my knees in prayer that very night, I begged God to look out after my wife and daughter and to protect them from my stupidity in choosing employers and from the likes of the "mean-shooter."

## CHAPTER 14

# MOVING TO GRANDMA'S GARAGE

WITH NO VIABLE PROSPECTS IN Chicago, a sawed-off shotgun slinger in our backyard and two fairly unpleasant experiences under my belt, I took my wife's counsel to move our things into Grandma's garage sixty miles east of St. Louis and try to find a job in the St. Louis area.

We rented a U-Haul truck and my Dad and teenage brother drove down from Chicago and helped us pack and move every non-breathing possession we had into Grandma's garage. Great Grandma was the best. She loved our daughter and enjoyed caring for her. She made us feel right at home and never asked for anything in return.

We liked our life there in my wife's hometown. With her parents nearby, lots of great things to do (like picking strawberries, harvesting and canning fresh vegetables from my in-laws' garden) and all the loving support we could tolerate, it was a refreshing time.

Since our student days in St. Louis, we had acquired a short-haired black (with brown accents) dachshund by the name of Kelsey. From baby Shannon's first day home from the hospital,

Kelsey thought our daughter was her own and seemed to take on this baby as her personal responsibility. Whenever we put Shannon down on the floor on a blanket, Kelsey would lie lengthwise on the border, getting up only to move closer if the baby rolled away. At Great Grandma's, Kelsey sat under the baby's highchair during meals and slept under her crib at nap-time and night-time. When Shannon was old enough to walk in the garden with Great Grandma, Kelsey was always close behind.

When I wasn't enjoying the good life with the family, I was busy calling everyone I knew to scare up a job somewhere in the vicinity.

In the meantime, we didn't lack for entertainment. There were church picnics, bingo nights and visits with friends around my wife's hometown to keep us busy and distracted from our worries.

At last, I contacted a former colleague, a graduate of St. Louis University's first class of P.A.s. Don was a twenty-year retired Army Master Sergeant. He had served in Korea and in Vietnam on two different tours. Thank God, he still clung to the paternal qualities that make Master Sergeants the kind of guys who can pull you through in a real pinch. And, when he heard about my situation, he promised an all-out effort to find an opportunity for me in St. Louis.

## CHAPTER 15

# THANK GOD FOR A POLISH WIFE

**M**ASTER SGT. DON PULLED THROUGH and leaked to me a rumor that the Department of Neurosurgery might be looking for someone. The first thing to do, he suggested, was to get our former Program Director, Dr. Frank, now the Medical Director of the V.A. hospital, to consider me as a viable applicant for any such position.

As the Program Director for the Physician Assistant Program, Dr. Frank (a man of Polish ancestry) was a tough task-master. He was the one who did final interviews with each applicant to the P.A. program. I had always respected him and liked him, but we had never had any one-on-one encounters so I had no way of knowing what his attitude might be toward me. Dr. Frank was an endocrinologist and a sharp doctor who had the respect of everyone in town. I didn't doubt that he had formed some opinion of me during my student years, he simply never had occasion to express it.

Without hesitation, I drove to St. Louis to meet with Dr. Frank in his office. Sgt. Don had paved the way for me. I knew he had made good on his promise when I walked into the administrative offices of the Veterans Hospital that morning and the secretary graciously invited me to have a seat. "The Director will see you shortly," she smiled.

Looking back on that day, I shudder to think how ill-prepared I was for such an important meeting, but I was confident that I had performed well in the program two years earlier and that my desire to succeed would carry me through. Sitting for almost an hour, I was more grateful for an audience than annoyed by the delay. Besides, it allowed me to ruminate – anxiously – over what I was going to say to convince this man to support my being hired into a system which, when compared to my experiences over the past couple of years, would surely be a haven.

The receptionist interrupted my thoughts with the invitation to go into Dr. Frank's office, "The Director is ready for you now." Seated in the big chair before his desk, I was alone just briefly before the connecting conference door opened and he entered, having obviously left a room full of people. I stood, we shook hands, and we sat down while Dr. Frank reached for his ever-present cigar. Lighting it, he looked up to say, "What brings you here?"

During the time I had known Dr. Frank, my female classmates had always regarded him as a teddy bear. Personally, I distanced myself from him. To me, he resembled a Kodiak bear, not the cozy, cuddly and pet-like companion the women saw, but one more threatening and wild-like. Consequently, I'm sure my voice lacked the strength of conviction I might have desired. Nevertheless, I recounted how I had spoken with Don and that I wanted to get to the front of any list of applicants, if it was true that a position might become available soon.

Dr. Frank was not very reassuring that any such position might open, but he did concede that there had been discussion of the matter. In what seemed to be a change of subject, he inquired about what I had been doing since I graduated from the program. That launched me into an account of my experiences to date, the details of which I had never intended to share, but Dr. Frank pulled the information out of me. His purpose, no doubt, was to discover what a graduate of the P.A. program he had created was actually experiencing out there in the real world. But, my fear was that he would think me a fool for getting into the circumstances that, one-by-one, I was persuaded to recount.

In his mind, this interview was a debriefing with a graduate and he took every advantage of the opportunity out of his love for the concept he had championed. From my perspective it felt more like an interrogation. More than an hour had passed when he finally noticed the time and leaned forward to remark that, while no decision had as yet been made about the position under discussion, he didn't think that it was going to happen in the immediate future.

Feeling almost desperate, I came to my feet and walked around from in front of his desk to approach him more directly. He swiveled his chair toward me as I knelt on my right knee and looked at him as penetratingly as possible. "Dr. Frank, please," I said. "No matter what you think of me, remember that my wife is Polish…and she and my little girl are depending upon your help as much as I am."

I quickly stood, shook his hand, thanked him for his time, and left his office.

CHAPTER 16

# WHAT MAKES YOU THINK YOU'RE QUALIFIED?

THE RIDE BACK "HOME" TO Great Grandma's that night was the longest sixty miles I can recall. My trip was a revolving rehash of the time I had spent in front of Dr. Frank – What had I said, what had I forgotten to say? Did I talk too much, too little? Did I present myself as worthy, or an idiot? Should I have knelt and said that thing about my Polish wife? I was tortured, and then it dawned on me: I didn't even give him my phone number or where I was staying. How could he reach me even if he wanted to?

As that thought surfaced, I rounded the corner at Great Grandma's and turned into her driveway. My headlights revealed the entire contents of our household, stacked to the ceiling on the right-hand side of the garage, which was clearly visible through the garage door windows.

Once inside, we sat together while I recounted the details of my meeting with Dr. Frank – many of which seemed ridiculous in hindsight – and my parting impulse was the crowning blow. But they both laughed, and somehow that made me feel better. At least they weren't gasping in horror at my impropriety.

The next morning I called the Master Sergeant Don and confessed the highlights of the prior day. He laughed too – long and loudly – but he also consoled me. According to him, Dr. Frank was more benevolent than not. He took down my phone number and promised to convey it to Dr. Frank. And with laughter still in his voice he excused himself to get on with his clinic duties. He promised a prompt call if he heard of any results from our efforts.

The following week I was amazed to get a call from him on a Friday evening. He was excited to announce that I had an interview with the Professor of Neurosurgery, Dr. Bill, the following Tuesday at 3:00 p.m. He wanted to know if I could be there. "Be there?" I shouted, "I'll leave now!" "No, no," Don laughed back, "just meet me in the clinic sometime around 2:00 p.m. and I'll take you up to meet him for the interview."

I was elated. I thanked my benefactor for his support and good will. We talked briefly about the uncertainty of it all but it was apparent that Dr. Bill had expressed an interest in meeting at the suggestion of Dr. Frank. It was clear that we were still a long way from reality, but, as Don suggested, it wouldn't hurt to get to know the man I might work for if it ever did happen.

Once off the phone I reported the details to my very patient wife and Great Grandma. The air was charged with a tentative enthusiasm that a job in this familiar community, not too far from my wife's family, might become a reality. My wife and her grandmother spent the next three days cajoling me not to use any outrageous tactics at the upcoming interview.

Tuesday came and I was out the door and down the highway well in advance of the necessary traveling time. Thoughts were racing through my head while I drove the familiar sixty miles past the famous St. Louis arch and onto Grand Boulevard toward the V.A. Hospital. Once inside, I met Don and was quickly ushered into a room where I sat on the far side of a small desk, face to face with Dr. Bill.

Dr. Bill was a full professor of neurosurgery at the Washington University School of Medicine. He had spent time in the military at the end of World War II, gaining great skills and camaraderie with the men and women of our armed forces. This led to a personal interest in the Veterans Administration hospital and although he never confided in me about this, I gathered from our conversation that his time there was a labor of love, more of a mission or a calling than anything else.

We talked for a long time. He asked me about my background and I asked him about his experiences and the breadth of his skills. Nothing of this interplay spoke of ego or braggadocio, and I was deeply impressed with this soft-spoken and gentle man.

We talked until the daylight faded into dusk. Finally, he looked me in the eye and asked quite frankly, "What makes you think you're qualified to do this?" I replied honestly. "I'm enthusiastic and willing to learn, and, if you're as good as you say you are, I'll know everything there is to know in no time at all!"

That brought a smile to his face. He shook my hand and said, "Well, you may be spending a lot of time in the library because I don't really know what you'll do, but we'll see what we can do about getting started."

CHAPTER 17

# ADVANCED NEUROSURGERY

T HE RIDE HOME TO GREAT Grandma's and the debriefing that followed was a joyous one. In the next few days we hopefully began to consider St. Louis our home, even though we knew we were counting our chickens a little prematurely. But, it wasn't long before we got another call from Master Sergeant Don saying that Dr. Frank wanted me to come to the Personnel Department ASAP and get the preliminary paperwork done. Thank God, our chickens had finally hatched!

I spent two days filling out government forms requiring endless detail about residences and references and finger-printing and on and on. Finally, I asked the personnel officer, "Why such an extensive paper chase?" "Top security clearance," he said. "Neurosurgery is where the President or Vice President could potentially be delivered for treatment in case of a medical emergency when they're in town so anyone who might be present, assisting or caring for a top government official has to pass top security clearance."

"No wonder they wanted me ASAP," I told my wife that night, "the paper work alone may take forever." But in two weeks I was duly processed and anxiously meeting my immediate supervisor, Dr. Shi. He had trained in neurosurgery at Washington University under Dr. Bill, and then left the U.S. to return home to Taiwan and practice after completion of his studies. Later, he and his wife came back to the United States to raise their family in St. Louis. However, the national board did not want to honor Dr. Shi's previous board certificate, as it had been granted without the written exam that was, at this time, a requirement. Had he stayed in the U.S., his certificate would have been grandfathered into the ranks when the written boards were instituted, but for now he was working at the V.A. and preparing to take the written boards.

The project proved to be no minor task for my mentor who, although multilingual, struggled with the nuances of Type K multiple choice tests that ask, "Which of these are true: A.) All of the above, B.) None of the above, C.) Items D and E, or D.) Items E and F." So, my first order of business was to promise to tutor Dr. Shi in the fine art of Type K question interpretation, and he promised, in return, to teach me everything he knew about neurosurgery.

This first day was – I remember well – a Friday, and his parting words to me were, "See you at crinic on Monday." I nodded, realizing I would have to learn some interpretative skills of my own in addition to my tasks at hand, but I was eager to do so.

Over the next few years, Dr. Shi became "Shi" and Dr. Bill became "Bill." They spent hours each week at patient bedsides, in the operating room and in classrooms on our floor teaching me their art – their love. Learning neurosurgery was a labor of love for me, too, as my contributions as a P.A. became a reality before the eyes of all three of us. It wasn't long before my presence was no longer an option, but a necessity. Bill went to bat to get me overtime pay so that I would be able to be at the hospital whenever I was needed, which turned out to be whenever either one of them was working.

Gone were the musings that I might have to spend my days in the library. Shi seemed to enjoy my company as much as I did his and we went everywhere in the hospital together. Each patient was another opportunity for him to teach me something, a lesson which would likely show up on the blackboard later that day in a neuroanatomy or neurophysiology lecture generated by the new consults we had seen.

Teaching rounds, journal articles and endless copies of Xeroxed text were ferried to me by these two brilliant surgeons with an intensity that surpassed even my heavily tutored days on Division II Medicine years before. But, I savored the learning as much as they did the teaching. My mind was a sponge and they enjoyed the friendly competition of filling up those interstices of my mental fiber with more and more of what they both so dearly loved.

## CHAPTER 18

# SAVED BY A BROOM IN
# A SNOW STORM

I N MY FIRST YEAR THERE, I was astonished by what an ordeal the neurosurgeon had to face in caring for patients. Neurosurgery is an extremely sophisticated skill that is hard-won over a seven-year residency. Nevertheless, the grunt work required to get to a decision to operate is further overshadowed by the pre-op processes of putting the patient on the table, arranging the instruments, sleeping the patient, positioning the patient and prepping the area before the operation.

Beyond that there was extensive traveling between centers for CT scans and the hassle of cumbersome angiograms. We had to do these ourselves by directly puncturing the carotid artery and filming on literally hundreds of film pieces which flashed continuously past a rapid-fire x-ray tube while we pushed dye into the patient's artery. Time and again we re-shot one view after another, only to discover that the "changer" had jammed, skipped or run out of film.

I timed hundreds of craniotomies. Once the patient was on the table, the surgery preparations took a minimum of two hours. It was not unheard of to take four hours just to do the incision, not to mention how long it took to saw through the skull with burr holes and giggly saws. This developed in me a quality of patience which I would not have suspected myself capable of developing, but I knew it was simply the minimum requirement for being there.

It was 4:30 one afternoon when we were called in for an emergency consult. The patient was a man who had been given a myelogram of his entire spine with an oil-based dye a few days earlier. Since then, he had become paralyzed from the neck down. A spinal tap conducted earlier that day was suggestive of meningitis (high white cell count and low spinal fluid glucose level).

Shi and I went to the floor to see the patient. We reviewed the chart, the laboratory reports and the films acquired during the myelogram – now 72 hours earlier. We re-examined the patient again some two or three hours later. As Shi looked at me through his full-lens reading-strength glasses, I was moved by this small man with such a great big heart, an even bigger mind and the largest eyeballs of any mammal known to man. Shi was severely nearsighted and wore bifocals outside the hospital, but at work he wore full-lens reading glasses with a resultant bug-eyed look that became his trademark.

"No choice," he said, "have to operate." Our work began. The skills I had developed – drawing bloods, filling out forms, and persuading staff by tugging at their heartstrings – were in full operation as I prepped the patient with up-to-date labs, blood bank samples and permits. I begged the O.R. supervisor to get our case on the schedule and I cajoled the tech in the blood bank to type, cross and set up four units of packed red blood cells immediately. I negotiated with the

Chief of Anesthesiology to provide the best possible anesthesia staff so we could perform a face-down (prone position) cervical-thoracic and lumbar spine decompression on a 300-pound man to save his spinal cord and (we hoped) restore his ability to walk and use his arms again.

Hours later we cut skin. The incision was in excess of 36 inches. The field was draped off with sterile towels firmly sutured into place, the skin edges retracted by large self-retaining rake-like tongs, exposing the entire length of the patient's spinal cord. The central nervous system is made up of the brain and spinal cord, and beyond the confines of its waterproof covering, lie the peripheral nerves. At the end of the spinal cord, which is usually at the level of the first two lumbar vertebrae, the bundle of nerves that go on to control the pelvis, bowel, bladder, legs and feet hangs freely in the spinal canal as the cauda equina (horse's tail). That covering of the spinal cord is called the duramater and is made up of three layers, collectively called the meninges. In this approach, we carefully incised the entire length of the waterproof layer from the top of the spinal cord to the lumbar spine.

Normally, the duramater is pink and relatively relaxed, but in this case the tissues were cherry red, shiny and tense as though inflated from within. The inner structures were encased in mucopurulent material that we cultured at multiple levels by gently teasing the pus-like accumulations off the surface of the spinal cord. Shi had confided in me in the locker room pre-operatively that he really didn't think the man was infected. If he were, the extent of his deficits and the time since the myelogram without diagnosis or the benefit of antibiotics would almost surely have killed him. Shi was convinced that the man had an almost equally sinister non-bacterial inflammatory response to the oil-based dye, triggered during the myelogram. He believed our patient to be the most unfortunate exception in medical history to have sustained the unheard-of response that we were witnessing.

Many hours later, after we had successfully re-closed the dura, achieved hemostatsis of all bleeders, closed the muscle, fascia and three layers of skin with interrupted sutures, we were able to turn him onto a stretcher and wake him up. We moved him into the ICU where we painstakingly recorded the details of the operation (Shi by dictaphone in a Chino-American dialect, and me by hand in the post-op note), and stood by our man until he recovered safely.

Post-op orders included broad spectrum high-dosed IV antibiotics, with Shi making the point that I must carefully check his cultures with the micro lab personnel in person each day. He emphasized that as soon as we could be assured that no organisms were present, we would be safe in utilizing high dose steroids to counteract the suspected inflammatory reaction.

We finally emerged from the front door to depart for home sometime around 2:00 a.m. and were startled by the wintry scene before us. Since last we had viewed the out of doors, six to eight inches of fresh snow had covered the earth and everything upon it. Shi quickly turned the corner to hop into his car while I trudged on through the thoroughly virgin blanket, my pant legs and shoes quickly encrusted in a frosty outer layer. My car, a used four-door Pontiac Bonneville once owned by my father-in-law, was literally buried under the thick blanket across the street about a block east at the very back of the parking lot annex. At this hour it was the only vehicle on the lot. Access to the lot was only partially restricted by sparsely placed swags of chain strung between loop-topped pipes driven into the asphalt and tipped in a wide variety of positions by any number of parkers past.

Reaching the rear of the car, I realized I had no ice scraper for the windows, and a thorough cleaning would be essential for the long trip home to Great Grandma's house. But I had stashed a corn broom in the trunk and I thought that should work. Sweeping the snow off the large trunk lid with my bare hand, I made a note to self: "Gloves, good purchase, as soon as possible."

I retrieved the broom and, in the sacred silence that characterizes such a snowy night, began pushing the blanket off in layers that seemed almost to be replaced before I could finish.

Suddenly I was aware of something. It might have been a barely perceptible crunchy squeak of snow underfoot, but whatever it was I heard or felt caused me to pause in my task for a microsecond and instinctively turn to face a thin, but tall man running directly at me. There was no thought, only the force of instantaneous anger exploding in me as I wound the broom at full backswing over my right shoulder, screaming, "I'll kill you, you son of a bitch," and bringing it down full force across his face.

The blow was superhuman for me, and my attacker was on his back struggling to get up while I stood straddling his legs and bludgeoning his form which was rolling about in the snow. The whole head of the broom released at this point and when I saw the handle – now broken into a lance-like point – I fully intended, in my abject panic, to impale him. Perceiving that, my would-be attacker somehow escaped the final blow, jumping to his feet and running off into the night without ever uttering a sound.

I stood shaking in the cold air, my hands encrusted with frozen snow, my broom disabled by the fray. I didn't notice the temperature or the time as I hurriedly cleaned the car and drove away toward the highway, my wife and my girl baby. Waves of gratitude rushed through me, as I realized I'd survived yet one more impediment to becoming the husband and father I so wanted to be. And, it occurred to me for an ironic instant that, only minutes after passionately trying to save a man's life and ability to walk, I had almost killed another with a broom handle.

Driving a car at eighty miles an hour in very snowy conditions requires a great deal of concentration. Thankfully, it can rid the mind of all else.

## CHAPTER 19

# A FIVE STAR HERO AND HEROIN

T HE RAVAGES OF WAR ARE almost inconceivably all-encompassing. The men and women who go off to defend our nation and our ideology of democracy and peace are far more important to you and me than any of us imagine. Their pain is often borne for a lifetime, and perhaps for generations, by those to whom they return when day is done.

Mickey had been a Green Beret in Vietnam, an extremely successful war-machine made of flesh and blood, heart and soul, mind and body. Decorated with five silver stars in combat, his personality and penchant for ruthless pursuit of the enemy took him to places most of us would never enter. When I met him, there was no reflection of any of these characteristics. He seemed as goodhearted and likeable as any other chap, but Mickey had a deeper problem.

While in South Vietnam, Mickey had acquired a sizable heroin habit that shaped his life and those around him. A regular at the "cleaners" in the Vietnamese village near his base, he dealt with the entrepreneurial proprietor, who not only cleaned clothes and did laundry for the men and women of our armed forces nearby, but also dabbled in the trafficking of narcotics to those who were so inclined.

At some point, Mickey and his "pusher" experienced a falling out over the quality of the "laundry." Mickey apparently killed the man, and as a result of the investigation that followed, he lost the job he loved and was sent back home.

It appears that the intelligence community was aware of the problem and had plans to eliminate the "dealer," but Mickey beat them to the punch, so to speak. So, while he incurred no direct punishment, he did get sent home. His addiction, of course, was sent home with him, and he became "employed" in the community, gaining sedation for his underground rage through more of the same.

Eventually, he met a similarly entrapped soul whose habit rivaled his. They married, and Mickey coerced her into prostitution as a source of capital for their unhappy dependency, until he got sick from his lifestyle and landed in our E.R. late one afternoon.

Recognized as one of the many like veterans who returned from "Nam" with a monkey on his back, and further informed by his mate, we scooped him up for the ride across town to the CT scanner at the university. It was there that we discovered a frontal brain abscess and significant edema surrounding it, so I got on the phone to arrange another emergency craniotomy and ICU bed reservation. Meanwhile, my Taiwanese colleague and attending physician made suggestions as to how we should approach the lesion surgically.

Through the night we toiled with the business at hand, and, with some medical pride (laced strongly with fatigue), we wrapped up the operation, bedded him down in ICU and

I headed for home – many hours too late for our daughter's grade school assembly that I'd promised to attend.

Weeks went by while we treated our hero with intravenous antibiotics in the hospital. Soon, we all had become a part of our patient's marital issues and his wife's pregnancy. She delivered a son shortly after Mickey's surgery and spent every day at the hospital with the infant in arm. I say "in arm" intentionally, as years earlier, during a drug induced stupor, she had slept on her arm, impairing her circulation to the limb for so many hours that she suffered a condition called a Volkmann's Ischemic Neuropathy and Contracture. That is, her left arm was limp and withered and her left hand was contracted into a fist-like deformity that rendered it useless.

Her heroin habit, curtailed by her husband's absence and the newborn baby's presence, made her a daily consumer of as much Valium as she could obtain to stave off her withdrawal discomfort between sparse "fixes." This behavior presented the entire staff with the dilemma of how to help this woman and her child. Night after night she dozed off in the dayroom which served as a visitors' parlor to the patients and their families on the floor. Other patients repeatedly alerted the nurses, as she fell asleep with the infant in her one functional hand, causing them to fear the baby would be dropped.

Our nurses and staff were a giving and self-sacrificing lot. They took the initiative and organized food, clothing, a baby bed, money and loving support for the woman and her child. They even took turns shuttling the infant to the nurses' station, ostensibly to change him, but often bathing and clothing him as well.

WHERE DO DOCTORS HIDE THEIR WINGS?

Finally, when they could no longer bear the drama of the young mother, they called Child and Family Services for assistance. The child was removed from the environment, and the parents were angry with the staff for their interference. Fortunately, though, the time had come for Mickey's discharge and they departed, leaving the rest of us hopeful that somehow they would be able to put things back together.

Months later, our nurses heard the news that Mickey and his wife were involved in an altercation on the steps of Valley Hospital late one night. For reasons we will never know, Mickey strangled and killed his wife in full view of witnesses who had called the police early in the argument.

Mickey was arrested and charged with murder, which he admitted to the judge openly, and was sentenced to prison for two years. At the end of two years, he was back out on the streets and came to see me at the clinic shortly thereafter.

I cannot forget that day. I was surprised to see him and didn't hesitate to ask if it was true that he had killed his wife. He acknowledged the fact and then announced that he was there because he had just been hit by a city bus two hours earlier. He demanded a prescription for Tylenol #3 with codeine. I explained that I could not write such a prescription – only the doctor had that prerogative – but even if I could, I would not. Angered, he jumped to his feet and stood in front of me announcing that he had a .357 magnum in his pocket and threatening to kill me too, on the spot.

I responded loudly that I wasn't going to take that type of behavior from him, either in threat or reality. "I gave up a lot for you to help save your life at the expense of my own family," I shouted, "Now, get out, and never come back unless you learn how to behave toward someone without the threat of violence." Underneath, of course, I was afraid, but my anger and expletives apparently demonstrated my resolve. He silently turned and walked out of the clinic, never to return.

## CHAPTER 20

# TOM AND HIS FRONTAL LOBES

I N THE LATE SEVENTIES AND eighties, medicine was frequently caught between the horns of a dilemma. No matter what unfortunate events befell our fellow citizens, whenever they lacked the wherewithal to pay for medical services, they were usually remanded to teaching institutions for care. This was particularly true of veterans.

Once someone determined that this particular unfortunate who lay in the local emergency room was once in the active duty armed forces, they were shipped, forthwith, to the nearest "Spa" hospital.

I will say that, in my twelve years of experience with that system, such a transfer – while it might seem to be a treatment reserved for second class citizens – was actually the best thing that could have happened to them. Centers such as ours were staffed by the very best medical minds and most dedicated students and residents under the supervision of the most sophisticated medical professors in the world.

One such young man had been out in the tall corn off a country road one sunny day in southern Missouri with his girlfriend. At the end of their picnic, they got into his pick-up truck and drove through the cornfield back to the road. They turned left onto the blacktop, only to be broadsided on the driver's side by an unsuspecting oncoming eighteen wheeler.

The girl was unhurt, but the driver, a barber from the "boot heel" of Missouri, was evacuated to us via ambulance. Arriving hours later, we identified his cervical spine fracture dislocation, a left complete pneumothorax and multiple lesser but unpleasant lacerations and contusions. Our team took the patient, stretcher and all, to the radiology department. Examined and x-rayed from head to toe within minutes, he was placed in traction tongs, his dislocation was reduced and the pneumothorax was identified.

Ninety minutes after his arrival we had him in traction in a bed on the fifth floor ward, and our general surgery residents from Unit I were there with us to decide the treatment plan for the patient's collapsed lung.

The patient was prepped, draped and scrubbed and the Chief Resident was poised to open the space between the man's 4th and 5th ribs to gain access for a chest tube. It suddenly dawned upon him that the patient was awake and no anesthetic had been administered. "Get me some lidocaine to numb him up – Quickly!" he barked authoritatively. "No need," we replied, "he's paralyzed and anesthetic from the neck down." The startled physician looked up with knife in hand to reveal his terror (and a wet eye) before proceeding silently.

Another young man arrived with a similar background from a rural portion of Missouri west of us. Tom had been involved in a head-on collision while driving on a two-lane road during an era long before airbags and the consistent use of seat belts.

In circumstances just like those of our barber friend, Tom arrived by ambulance critically injured, comatose and with a bone-exposing forehead laceration and a fractured skull that extended from sideburn to sideburn. With the help of every nurse in our emergency room, we cut off his clothes, washed his blood-soaked body from head to toe and dressed his head wound with the typical neurosurgeon's turban while awaiting the ambulance to ferry us to the only EMI CT scanner in the city.

Still hours later, we returned and bedded him down in our ICU. Our attending professor arrived unannounced to examine the youth and determine the plan for his care. Dr. Bill was a great neurosurgeon and combat-experienced. He knew intimately the care of such massive head trauma and he gladly took the opportunity to teach as he worked to examine our patient.

Dr. Bill discussed the options openly and advised that we had no recourse but to operate on Tom right then and there, which created a flurry of events too convoluted to relate here. One had to be a multi-tasking expert to obtain the necessary consent for surgery from his mother, prepare a space on the schedule in the operating room, obtain blood samples for type and cross (the minimum was four units – this day we asked for six), and on and on.

Dr. Bill went back to the university hospital for evening rounds on his patients there, returning three hours later to join us in the operating room where we had already opened a bi-frontal craniotomy. That was my first experience of freeing the upper face from the skull and facial bones in order to peel it forward all the way to the tip of the nose.

After hours of tedious coagulation and careful decompression of blood clots from Tom's two frontal lobes, Dr. Bill quietly remarked how we had no choice. "If we close the head and leave all this contused brain, he will certainly herniate from the swelling and die." The alternative then occupied another three or four hours, while we painstakingly resected both frontal lobes, achieved hemostasis, and closed the meninges, layer after layer, until we could unwrap the upper third of his face and suture it back into place.

The night ended with post-op notes, orders and bedding the patient down in ICU. Since it was too late to drive back home, I slept on the treatment table back on the fifth floor for about ninety minutes before the change of nursing shifts drove me from my mat. The morning, full of rounds and consults, was no impediment to our plans for Tom on the floor below in ICU. The lone CT scanner would not be vacant until 4:00 p.m. that day and we had already arranged another ambulance and the trip for a post-op scan that night.

After weeks of coma and daily trips – times many – to the ICU, my Taiwanese mentor remarked that "thirteen is the magic number."

"What's that supposed to mean?" I asked.

Dr. Shi answered, "More than thirteen weeks in coma, and he may never wake up."

But as the magic number neared, Tom began to wake up, albeit slowly. His recovery was delayed further by a bone flap infection that required removal of all the devitalized bone we had cut from his skull that first night. Weeks more of intravenous antibiotics and our young man healed, but with the absence of his bony forehead. It was unsightly and would have drawn stares and unwanted attention in any other environment, but not from these comrades, already hardened by the sight of even more nightmarish war wounds.

Eventually, we repaired even his cosmetic defects successfully, and he returned home. His personality and behavior, however, had been altered and it was no surprise to those of us on the fifth floor. We had gotten used to Tom's new habits of insatiable eating and lusty staring at our nurses. At first, I was puzzled by his behavior, but my mentor took the observations I shared with him as a perfect opportunity to lecture me on the anatomy and function of the brain. He included laboratory observations of previous and similar behavioral changes that followed the destruction or removal of the frontal lobes.

It seems that one of the major roles of the frontal lobes involves filtering one's affect and mood, including the desire for food and sexual gratification. Tampering with those filters, then, had predictable results. That said, you might not be surprised that once he was discharged and home again, Tom experienced repeated encounters with the community and legal system in his rather rural community. On four occasions, a local judge contacted me, asking for an explanation of Tom's surgery and its possible effect on his behavior. In every instance, the offense was relatively harmless and the community was more embarrassed than anything else.

Tom was a regular in my clinic and came for follow-ups every six months. On one such visit, he proudly showed me photographs of his girlfriend and informed me of their mutual proclivity for very frequent intimacy. He announced he was going to marry her, and sure enough, six months later he arrived with his bride in tow. She was very nice, and there was an obvious attraction between them, which in her presence, Tom graphically described. I pleaded out of the more lurid details on the grounds that I had so many patients I had to see that day.

In parting, I sincerely wished them happiness and watched as they walked away together. I never saw either of them again. And I never received another call from a judge in the matter of Tom's behavior. I like to think that they lived happily ever after.

## CHAPTER 21

# A QUAD CAN'T PULL
# THE TRIGGER

NOT EVERY DAY WAS QUITE SO emotionally packed, thank God. Most of the time, the V.A. was a great place to be. There was an underlying stream of kindness that seemed to guide everyone in that environment, and I was aware early on that if I focused on that and asked anyone for assistance they would immediately respond and participate in whatever cause was at hand.

We laughed together, cried, sang, ate and worked side-by-side. We all shared a deep appreciation and sense of responsibility for these fallen men and women. Our particular floor was home to Neurosurgery, Surgical Oncology and Plastic Surgery meaning our patients were some of the worst injured, mutilated and incapacitated. As a result, our nurses, aides and techs were often overwhelmed emotionally by caring for them. Noticing this, I took it upon myself to consult with both the chaplain and psychiatrist regarding many of the patients and the staff who cared for them.

Eventually, the psychiatrist, Sidney, agreed to conduct private one-hour sessions every thirty days with our staff to re-center our thoughts and reinforce our awareness of the value of our work with the patients, in spite of the overwhelming feelings we often experienced.

It was a great program, never officially documented nor discussed with Dr. Frank, but somehow I knew he knew and approved.

Our work became a topic of discussion about the time Shi was called to leave the U.S.A. and return to Taiwan. His father had been diagnosed with inoperable cancer, and, as the oldest son, it was up to Shi to take over the family businesses and his father's affairs. I knew he was disappointed because he had just reached the point where we both knew he could easily pass his boards. When I made that observation, his response was simple. "No choice," he said to me.

Shi's resignation led to a flurry of conference room consultations and I suspected that Bill and Dr. Frank were discussing what had just been scuttled by that turn of events. That same day Bill showed up on our floor, unannounced, and asked to speak with me. When he walked up to the nursing station and addressed our head nurse by name (she was shocked he even knew her name) and then asked for me specifically, she feared something was amiss.

But that was not the case. In the face of the changes, he wanted to reaffirm the importance and security of my position there. He assured me that if I remained he would afford me support from faculty until he could arrange resident coverage. He also suggested that a joint appointment with the Wash U. Medical School would likely be forthcoming, as well as a substantial increase in salary and benefits.

Frankly, I was elated to survive the departure of Shi, let alone be given the possibility of a Washington University

Medical School appointment and a promise of permanence. Nevertheless, as he shook my hand I had to quip (with tongue in cheek, of course), "Thanks Bill. I guess that means I won't be spending any more time in the library?"

Every day was a new experience for me. I was surrounded by men who had lived through WWII, as had my own Dad, my uncles and so many others. I walked the halls and asked questions, just as I had been taught, with remarkable results.

We were the first line evaluators of all military personnel with spinal cord injuries whose home or family was in our region. The nation has five such centers. Immediately upon evacuation to the U.S. from a war zone or foreign outpost, the newly injured are brought to the neurosurgery center in the region for evaluation, stabilization and referral to rehab. From early on, I was eager to get to know these men and women and basically learn how to understand them and be there for them.

One of my most immediate connections was with a young paraplegic fellow who had been injured in Vietnam. He was a regular on our service for plastic surgery and an occasional neurosurgery consult. Not too long into our friendship, I felt comfortable asking Mark to help me understand how patients with disabilities like his learn to cope. Seated in his VA-issued quickie wheelchair in my office, smoking a cigarette and enjoying my personal coffee stash, Mark began to talk. I listened for some time, and, as he lit another cigarette I asked pointedly, "Mark, what's the difference between a quadriplegic and a paraplegic?"

He looked up, stared at me somberly, and then softly remarked: "A quad can't pull the trigger."

CHAPTER 22

# GIVE ME YOUR PAIN

L IFE AT THE V.A HOSPITAL was not like anywhere else
I had been. The people who worked there were truly
special. They weren't without their gripes and faults,
but who among us is? Even though the sadness of our patients
and the degree of sickness and loneliness was sometimes
overwhelming for our staff, they came back to it day after day.
Sidney, my psychiatrist friend, was often found on the ward
talking to a patient about the sadness of his experiences in
wartime, and how that experience had fashioned his relation-
ships since coming home.

I never heard the vets actually discuss the reason for their
amazing sense of camaraderie, but I think I know. They
seemed to share a common thread that those of us who have
never had to face ourselves in war cannot imagine. Faced with
a "kill or be killed" situation, I suspect that most of us would
behave differently than we would like to imagine ourselves.
Soldiers have had to face a grim internal reality that cannot be
understood – let alone discussed – with wives, sons, daugh-
ters or even brothers.

They don't speak of their experiences with one another
either, but they seem to know what each of them has had to

come to grips with about themselves and can't express. The twelve years I spent with them left me with a deep respect for these mostly silent men and women and the strength of their bond.

Many of them had actually been surgically silenced. Suffering head and neck cancers from cigarette smoking, they had been through drastic surgeries that left them with no voice box and permanent tracheotomies. Nevertheless, most of them still smoked. During my time there, smoking was allowed in the hospital, although that is no longer the case.

I was standing in the corridor one day when one such patient came walking down the hall with his cigarette. Allow me to enlighten you about the process of smoking with a tracheotomy. One must hold the cigarette to one's lips while simultaneous blocking the opening to the windpipe with a finger from the opposite hand. Then, having inhaled the smoke, the patient can remove the occluding finger and exhale the smoke through the trach.

With that image in your mind, you can see what I observed as this fellow walked past me and encountered another patient laying on a stretcher across the corridor. Without a word, the chap took the cigarette from his own lips and stopped to hold it to the lips of the man on the stretcher, who took a drag himself. Then the walker – still silent – put the cigarette to his own lips again and walked on.

These many years later, I still wonder at that intimacy – that bond, or brotherhood – they all share. It's no wonder that we hear today of men and women who suffer the injuries of war and yet are seen to cry openly when faced with the reality that they will be sent home for good, leaving their colleagues behind to fight on without them. It is just this bond that I observed, day in and day out. I became acutely sensitive to the way they shared each others' suffering. They grieved whenever one of them worsened and was moved from the ward to one of the twelve private rooms down the hall from the nurses' station. The men called it "death row," and, when one of them was transferred to a private room on that hall, they would find a means to visit their comrade, one way or another.

Those who could walk would push those who could not, in wheelchairs or on stretchers, and they would stand outside the private room and talk to the vet within, day after day, until he was no longer there. And these were people who had never served together; in fact, it's likely they had never met at all before arriving at the V.A. (or the "Spa" as they called it). But their camaraderie required no introductions. They took up with one another instantly and looked out for each other just the same.

There was one particular experience that pierced my soul. Interviewing newly admitted patients was a daily routine for me. It took place right there on the ward, with the new patient and me separated from those around us only by a curtain hanging from an aluminum track above each bed. On this occasion I was taking a history from a nineteen-year-old Marine who'd done his boot camp in California little more than six weeks earlier. In celebrating their graduation from boot camp, my patient and a young Latino soldier he'd met in basic training, went to the beach to see the ocean for the first time. They put their towels on the sand, rubber-necking to take in the varied beauty of the female scenery, and my patient decided to jump up and try out the salt water.

As I interviewed the young man, asking question after question, a potent silence surrounded us, caused by the listening of the other patients, who were separated from our awareness only by the thin fabric surrounding our position in the center of the ward. As the young man relived the horror of the events that had brought him to this place, his voice began to crack. He related how the six foot waves had floated his feet off the sandy bottom, and how one particular wave had completely upended him and thrust his body head-first into the depths, severing his spinal cord and leaving him helpless.

Now, lying motionless on his back, tears welled up and he recalled the bubbles of his last breath as he helplessly awaited his own death. At apparently the same instant, his Latino friend sat up, as though alerted by a sense of danger. When he realized his fellow Marine was not in sight, he sprang to his feet and dashed into the ocean screaming his buddy's name. Diving into the surf, again and again, he searched the blue-green foam until he found him. He pulled his comrade to safety and dragged his limp body up the beach to the clamor of lifeguards who rushed to assist him.

My patient, now crying openly, having finished his tale, began to sob, "It hurts too much, my neck, it hurts!"

Suddenly, the stillness around us was broken by a loud voice crying out from the bed next to us in a voice that could no longer remain silent. "Give *me* your pain. *Give me your pain!*"

## CHAPTER 23

# TRAVELING TO THE SACRED PLACE, THE SEAT OF THE SOUL

T RADITIONALLY, SURGEONS HAVE REGARDED THE operating room as a sanctuary, a place of solitude and silence. Most of the more experienced surgeons with whom I studied used little or no verbal communication during surgery, and many used only hand signals to ask for a particular instrument. It seemed to me to be particularly true of neurosurgeons for whom maximal concentration and focus were essential to the success of the operation. No one dared to tell jokes, laugh or bang instruments during this time. It was only the surgeon who was allowed to have outbursts of any kind.

Dr. Bill was a classic for this, and only upon the occasion of an aneurysm surgery would he, almost ceremoniously, kick the wheeled stainless steel bucket (appropriately called the kick bucket). During twelve years and countless surgeries, before we cut skin on an aneurysm case, something inevitably would be out of place or missing, and Dr. Bill would mutter loudly and kick the bucket. It would skid across the terrazzo floor, hit the wall and fly upward about three feet before crashing to the floor with a resounding clatter. I became convinced that this was a kind of release from the gut-wrenching tension, as well as a last minute way to gain the undivided attention of everyone in the room.

Whatever it was, it worked. Each and every one of us would be absolutely silent and on pins and needles as the tedious work of isolating, meticulously dissecting and clipping the aneurysm was accomplished. I learned early in my neurosurgery career that time was not of the essence and any attempt to plan or anticipate the time of our emergence from the O.R. was futile.

On one such occasion, we undertook the surgical removal of a third ventricle aqueduct tumor by entering from below and following the aqueduct rostrally from within the fourth ventricle. Since that jargon is foreign to most of you, let me explain. The ventricles are like cisterns within the deepest recesses of the brain. They are filled with a water-like fluid called cerebro-spinal fluid, which is non-cellular blood serum that is clear and colorless and contains oxygen and glucose to feed the brain from within.

At a juncture where the brain and the brainstem transition, the fourth ventricle is the last of the series and feeds spinal fluid to the central canal of the entire spinal cord below. The third ventricle is rostral (toward the top of the head) to the fourth, and this approach takes the surgeon quite literally to the center of the brain.

I felt a strange sense of wonder as I gazed into this sacred space, where no sound had ever penetrated and which no human eye had ever seen. It was a silent and breathtakingly awesome experience, this penetration into the center of human awareness. My thoughts were so overwhelming that it was moments before I suddenly became aware of my need to breathe. In that sacred silence I became utterly convinced that we had been allowed to see the very seat of the soul.

Remarkably, we were successful in removing the tiny obstructing tumor without apparent harm to the surrounding tissue and some two weeks later, the man walked out the front door of the hospital into the warm St. Louis sunshine.

## CHAPTER 24

# DEPRESSION AND HIS WIFE'S PET PIG

B ECAUSE OF THE HOSPITAL'S LOCATION within the city and its juxtaposition to the housing across the street, crime was a way of life outside the fence surrounding this federal reserve. Within the boundaries, security was more than adequate, but outside that fence, look out. The biggest problem we had was coming and going after dark and before daylight, and it was even worse when the New Year's holiday came upon us. Annually, the Chief of Staff would issue a directive that on New Year's Eve between the hours of 11:00 p.m. And 1:00 a.m. we were not to attempt to enter or leave the premises. During my twelve years there, two employees who failed to heed the 11:00 p.m. to 1:00 a.m. directive were shot (albeit not fatally) in an attempt to go through the front doors of the hospital.

Furthermore, the twelve rooms that the patients referred to as Death Row had to be cleared on that night. The nurses rolled all the beds into the interior corridors and away from the front windows of the building, because, as midnight approached, the city would explode with fireworks and firearms throughout the area. The nurses were dutiful about the care of the patients, and, although some light bulbs and windows were shattered on occasion, no one had ever been hurt inside the building.

It was not on New Year's Eve, but during the Christmas holidays (when more people experience depression than any other time of the year) that I was called to the Emergency Room at 11:30 p.m. I jumped in the car and headed into the city with dispatch, as my resident had spoken urgently and seemed anxious that I get there as soon as possible. Dr. Keith was convinced that surgery was necessary but we would first have to ferry the patient to the university for an EMI CT scan.

I drove pedal to the metal and turned off the highway onto Grand Boulevard at an equally rapid pace. When I came to a red light (it seemed as if all of them were red that night), I laid on the horn and drove straight through. Actually, it was always my habit to drive through the red lights on the way to the hospital, since coming to a complete stop in that section of town could prove fatal. Certain citizens had a habit of using baseball bats to smash the driver's side window at a stoplight and rob him or her. The regulars at the hospital who worked nights carried a .38 in their pockets when going in at night, and many of the night nurses carried .32s in their purses for similar reasons.

In any event, I got to the parking lot inside the iron fence and adjacent to the E.R. in almost no time at all. I parked and got out of the car, only to be greeted by a police officer with gun drawn and trained on me. My hands were up over my head in a micro-second, and apologies, laced with explanations about the emergency circumstances, poured out of my mouth.

Just then the ambulance we had summoned pulled into the area and the urgency of the situation was abundantly apparent. The policeman chastised me briefly, and I was penitent, but I pleaded "duty first."

The patient, the stretcher and my resident emerged from the E.R. We all loaded into the ambulance and raced off into the night, lights and sirens ablaze.

While the patient went through the ordeal of the scan, my colleague filled me in on the three weeks leading up to our patient's arrival from Elsewhere, Missouri. It seems we had treated this patient before, but he was never able to regain his ability to provide for his family. His wife and family became judgmental, and the patient fell into a severe depression, which he self-medicated with increasing amounts of alcohol. Ultimately, the fellow's family abandoned him, and finally, in desperation, his wife also took flight. Drunk most of the time, lonely and depressed, our patient had brought his wife's pet pig into the house to keep him company.

The pig made a mess of the house, which the depressed man did not bother to address, and by the time he was discovered, both he and the house were covered with filth. In the midst of the filth and chaos, the patient told us later, he had become even more despondent. In a fit of despair, he had set fire to the curtains, shot the pig and turned the pistol on himself, putting a .38 caliber bullet into his right temporal lobe. That was the state in which we found him.

After a lengthy and laborious craniotomy, the patient survived and a month later his wife and grown children came to the "Spa" to bring him home. The house had been saved by neighbors, scrubbed, and restored to its former condition.

The family was now back in their home, willing to forgive and put the tragedy behind them. Sidney, our psychiatrist, had been able to help the patient with his depression, and all was now well (except for the 450 pound pig, who was dead).

CHAPTER 25

# DO THINGS EVER CHANGE?

SOMEWHERE AROUND TEN YEARS INTO this frenetic pace, between living up to my promises to Dr. Bill and my intentions for those who trusted me with their lives, I began to get weary of the late nights and long hours at the hospital. A growing sense of family responsibility and a need to do the right thing for everyone's sake became paramount in my mind. Our daughter was nearing high school and had been playing violin since she was three years old. I had been a devoted father, but in absentia most of those years. In fact, my children would never have seen me except for the fact that my flexible wife insisted we all have dinner together, even though that rarely occurred before 9:00 p.m. She reasoned that it was better for children to know their father than to have a normal dinner and bedtime. For that I will be forever grateful.

During those ten years we scraped every chip of old paint off our house, twice. We repainted it inside and out and we built fences and bookshelves with the help of one of our residents and his wife, who became dear friends. I even helped him with projects such as a tanning bed and a complete tear-off and re-roof of his house (and I can tell you that is something I will never do again!). My time away from my family was beginning to gnaw at me. So, one day when a former resident whom I liked and respected called me from Atlanta, I was interested. "We need you here," he told me, "I want you to come and interview with my partners."

When the time is ripe for change, those are the words one longs to hear—the hopeful sound of opportunity calling. After a few telephone negotiations over the next two weeks, Peg and I had come to terms with the possibility of leaving. We agreed to come and look at what they had to offer. We were convinced that, if we were intended to move, the impediments would be lifted and everything would work out quickly.

Two trips to Atlanta, and we were packing to move into a gorgeous new home which fulfilled a long standing wish—it had more than one bathroom! We were thrilled. Atlanta was beautiful and held a promise for more time together, more money and the glamour of private practice.

Back in St. Louis I had the unenviable task of telling Dr. Bill that I was leaving. He so disliked that prospect that he came over to my office and spent an afternoon trying to talk me out of it. His very tone spoke volumes and I would like to think he was proud of what I had become in his shadow. He told me he planned to resign his attending position at the "Spa" and made it clear that his decision was predicated on my leaving. I viewed this development with a mixture of guilt and pride but, for better or worse, my own motivations were tied to the move and a better life for my wife and family.

Packing, listing the house and saying our goodbyes to friends and neighbors took some time, but before long we moved into our new home. The family was ecstatic. Personally, I admit to feeling undeserving of what seemed to me a veritable mansion compared to our previous surroundings. I think I never quite got used to it. Settling in was not without its issues, as they say, and two months had not passed before I was introduced to the real reason I had been selected for the post.

Prior to my joining the group, the practice had been in the habit of allowing office staff to cover prescription refill requests for patients. They diligently recorded every telephone call and had one of the physicians review the details, but somehow one particularly violent fellow had taken umbrage with a refusal for narcotic refills and pumped seven 30-06 slugs into the office/clinic one night after hours. Two shots fired from the deer rifle traversed the front wall of the building into the office of the founder and lodged in a bookcase. Two more entered the waiting room and the secretarial area. Three others went through two walls and a cabinet in the kitchen and lodged in the back wall of the building, a good fifty feet from the façade of the building.

Although that might have intimidated other possible P.A. candidates, it certainly did not scare me. After all, I had spent 12 years at the "Spa" where things like that were practically commonplace.

Here, in the fancy private offices of my new practice, with bullets lodged in several walls, I realized that perhaps I had simply jumped from the frying pan into the fire. Nonetheless, I felt right at home.

I guess some things just never change.

CHAPTER 26

# AN UNPAID BILL, A TRUCK, AND A YEAR OF MALE BONDING

ATLANTA WAS A WHOLE NEW world for all of us. "Adjusting" would be a word far too conservative to depict the changes and uncertainties that we experienced during that transition. The good news was that we worked with some really nice people and, although we had our ups and downs as we experienced one personal and family challenge after another, my work went to a new level of excellence and was very fulfilling.

Our patients and their families were most appreciative and our acceptance in the community was – although a mixed experience – in general, very affirming. Time and again detractors were pleasantly surprised by our effectiveness, and for the most part I was able to keep my employers satisfied.

The downside was that I now had three bosses and as my personal effectiveness became more apparent, their demand for my presence became even greater. A sort of tug-of-war regarding where and with whom I should be working gradually emerged and a measure of unhealthy paranoia crept under the door. Once again, I began to spend more and more time at work and less and less at home. In a few years, I had succeeded in escalating my work schedule to seven days a week, which was even more stringent than the schedule I'd kept in St. Louis. Eventually, I was honest enough to assess the situation. When I realized I couldn't really change the circumstances, I learned to change myself instead.

I grew a great deal during those days and began to enjoy the fruits of my ability to influence our patients' experiences and improve their outcomes with my positive input. One such opportunity involved a young man whom we'll call Tony. The fellow had a very bad back and was properly diagnosed with a ruptured lumbar disc, which ultimately resulted in surgery at the hands of one of my bosses. I assisted in the surgery and was a first-hand witness to a good operation with no breaks in sterile technique and no contributing misfortune.

His post-operative recovery was excellent early on, but an increase in his pain and a wound infection progressed into a severe disc-space infection. He was treated promptly and appropriately, but in the ensuing months his continued pain required another operation, which failed to rectify the scar tissue seen in the second procedure. From that point on, the surgeon was upset with his inability to mitigate the patient's pain, and he requested that I give special attention to this patient in follow-up and offer any reasonable treatment I could.

Pain medication in moderation, tri-cyclic antidepressants and regular follow-up appointments went on for almost a year. One day, the man came into the office for a follow-up appointment. When I asked him to schedule his next visit in six months, or sooner if needed, he protested. He got very quiet, and with some encouragement revealed that every appointment he attended was punctuated by a meeting with our accounts receivable collector who kept reminding him of his growing indebtedness of over $14,000. He was embarrassed and uncomfortable about not being able to pay the debt. He was a man of honor and hard working prior to his back surgery, but humbled by his disability and financial destitution.

Promising to review this with his doctor, and reassuring him that Dr. Greg and I would find a way to help him solve the dilemma, I encouraged him to schedule his next follow up appointment, and he departed. When Dr. Greg came into the office to do paperwork at the end of the day, I approached him with what had happened, and he expressed sympathy for the man. Then, he asked me what I thought we should do. I asked if we could forgive the debt, and if I could be permitted to see the patient at the same intervals for as long as necessary, but without levying a charge for any subsequent visits.

I was surprised at how quickly Dr. Greg agreed, and, later that very evening, a call to the patient to relay the doctor's generosity was greeted with great relief. This type of event became a regular scenario in our practice from that point on, amounting to easily thirty percent of our patients' unpaid bills. Despite the voluntary release of so many accounts receivable, the practice became more and more successful every year and the generosity of each doctor served to stimulate a similar generosity in the other two.

Months later, I got a call at the office from Tony, who invited me to come to his parents' home on Saturday. When I inquired as to the occasion, Tony said he had a pick-up truck that he could no longer drive because of his back pain, and he wanted to give it to me. I told him I didn't feel right taking anything from him, but he protested. He said the truck didn't run anymore (something about a broken timing chain), but he felt sure I could repair it. Even if I wouldn't take the truck, he wanted to give it to our son.

Our son, Joe, was still in elementary school. "Joe's just a kid, Tony," I said, "he can't even drive." But Tony would not take "no" for an answer. My wife pointed out that, while he couldn't give the truck to my boss, he felt he could do something for me. "He's just trying to thank you somehow," she said. "It's something you should let him do."

We agreed on a time and place to meet, and I drove out to tow the '68 Chevy pick-up back to our garage. For the next year, Joe and I pushed that truck out of our garage almost every Saturday and began to work on it. Our neighbor up the street, who loved doing this sort of thing, often waltzed down to join the two of us under the raised hood. "Hey, Joey," he would whisper, "how about getting me a beer?" And so the three of us would plan the next step of our year-long process.

The age of the truck left us without a manual, and our own lack of ingenuity took us to the auto parts store week after week, with various pieces in hand, asking what tool we might need in order to get over the present hurdle. No kidding, this was a real challenge. I had learned a few car things from my Dad as a boy, but my knowledge was minimal, and we had certainly never replaced a timing chain. Nevertheless, there's something about working on a car for a whole year with your son that can't quite be explained. "It's male bonding," my wife said. I suppose that's what our efforts were actually about. After all, I had been gone more than I had been home, so this old truck became the gift that brought my son and me together in a way nothing else could quite have done. Meanwhile, my wife and daughter watched us in the driveway each Saturday for what must have seemed to them like much longer than a year.

Finally, miraculously, it happened. After cranking the engine and searching desperately for that "sweet spot" on the spark advance by rotating the distributor clockwise and counterclockwise endlessly, she fired up! Straight dual pipes with minimal muffling from glass packs did little to diminish the roar of this huge eight-cylinder engine as it disrupted the ambiance of our prestigious subdivision.

Cheers of joy erupted from our little pit crew that day, and two of the three of us celebrated with another beer.

CHAPTER 27

# THE LAST PAYMENT

T HE TRUCK WAS A LANDMARK in our lives. From that point on, my daily work took on a new perspective, and, while not always noticed or appreciated, had been better intended.

Having proudly announced the resurrection of the white Chevy truck, Joe and I got repeated invitations to come out and visit Tony. On each visit he revealed more of his personal interests and hobbies. He was an outdoorsman, and somewhat of a naturalist. We found on one occasion that he had rescued an owl with a broken wing.

Tony was living with his grandmother, and like all grandmas, she felt that Tony could do no wrong. So she didn't object when he installed a substantial segment of a huge tree into the day room adjacent to the living room of the house. With the owl perched there on the tree, Grandma, grandson and their companion owl watched television in bliss and friendship. Since the owl required a mouse or two for sustenance, a significant mess was continually present, but it didn't seem to bother Grandma.

I think the owl liked his new home because even when he was fully healed and quite able to fly about, he never tried.

Nevertheless, a neighbor apparently called the Humane Society and reported the captive creature and Tony was forced to release his feathered fellow back into the woods.

Tony's (and Grandma's) home was surrounded by trappings of his special relationship with nature, sport and hunting. One of his avocations was raising Plott Hounds, a special breed of dog from the back hills of North Carolina with a genetic talent for tracking and hunting wild boars and bears.

On one of our trips to see Tony, he introduced us to his Plott Hounds. The male was massive. He was tethered to a tree with a long chain while the female had free rein of the property as she herded her little pups around the yard. A powerful and very aggressive breed, this dog has no apparent fear when confronted with a bear, a trait that I confess I found impressive.

Some months later, Tony called me at home. It happened to be a rare evening when I had come home from the office at a decent time. He asked for directions to our house, stating that he and his Mom wanted to drive over and bring something to our son. I inquired what they had in mind, and once again reiterated that he need not continue to give us things. He said he knew that and acknowledged my feelings, but he insisted that he must come over and refused to divulge the reason for his visit. He simply said he would be there in an hour.

Joe was twelve or thirteen years old, and I vividly recall my own surprise when Tony stood at the door as I opened it. It was a cold, gray winter day in Atlanta, and wrapped within his arms, snuggled against his jacket, was a little ball of black-brindle fur. Tony walked into the family room where

Joe was lying on the floor watching television and he put the puppy down on the carpet.

She headed straight for our son and began biting at his hair and pulling at it playfully. Within seconds they were rolling about the floor – instant friends – and their joy filled our hearts. Tony beamed, as did I. We all thanked him for the gift, and for his willingness to make the trek across town to deliver her. Tony, his well-guarded emotions very near the surface, shook my hand and remarked, "It was my pleasure." Without another word, and before the tears could actually fall, he turned quickly and went out the door, his Mom close behind.

The season was Christmas and the pup's brindle coloration prompted our daughter, Shannon, to suggest the name, Chestnut. We knew that Chessie was a final and very heartfelt payment of love from a man who had become much more than a patient to all of us.

Chessie is an old dog these days. Her chestnut fur is turning gray around her eyes, reminding us that time marches on. But she is a cherished member of our family and a vivid reminder of why we came to Georgia – a reminder of what, at its core, the practice of medicine is all about.

# THE REASONING
# BEHIND THIS BOOK

AT THIS POINT IN THE completion of this work, I am besieged by those who have inquired as to what prompted me to take my laptop in hand, so to speak, to pen my thoughts. In a task much more difficult than what it may seem, I have had to retrospectively examine what I am saying in contradistinction to what might be common knowledge, or at least what too many of my patients might see as lacking in medicine this day in age.

I decided that my immense respect for physicians as acquired over the decades is based in an intimate knowledge of their humility and a thankless desire to restore all their patients to health, in spite of the brutal reality that even Herculean efforts are oft met with disappointment.

I have felt the intensity of their heartfelt efforts and experienced the depth of their despair as they grappled with their limitations. It is ultimately that breech between initiation and successful completion that must be reconciled by the physician and his or her patient to reach resolution.

That's right! A book to begin a conversation – a dialogue between patients who need super human efforts to restore their well being and a practitioner who will be capable of exceptional levels of success. If you are thinking that it is not the book itself that the reader should revere, but the conversation between the patient and the physician, you are precisely correct!

There is an approach to initiate this conversation in one's search for the "right one" to accept the task ahead. It requires a cognizance of this book and its contents on the part of patient and practitioner alike. Not only does the patient have to speak the words, but they must, in turn, be recognized by the listener.

Simply, entreat the practitioners with the plea..."Please – show me your WINGS!"

*-Dennis*

# EPILOGUE

What lies before us and
What lies behind us are
Tiny as compared with what
Lies within us
*-Emerson*

# Glossary

ANASTAMOSE – Surgically connect two segments of tissue as in connecting the free ends of the colon after a partial resection

CEPHALIC – A description of that area that represents the head or in the direction of the top of the head

CERVICAL-THORACIC DECOMPRESSIONS – Removing the bony element of the vertebrae to relieve spinal cord compression

CREATININE – A measure of the kidney's function, the serum creatinine is most accurate

EMI CT SCAN – Another term for the Magnetic Resonance Imaging of the human body that does not use x-rays and is more sensitive

ENDOCRINOLOGIST – A medical specialist in Endorinology, as in the glandular systems such as the pancreas or adrenal glands that affect

ETIOLOGY – The physiologic cause of a condition

FASCIA – A connective tissue layer that maintains separation and containment

GIGGLY SAW – A handheld mechanical saw that has removable handles and is similar to a flexible cable, has coarse spurs protruding from the cable allowing one to slide the saw under the skull through "burr holes" and place the handles on each end and lift. A to-and-fro motion causes the saw to cut the bone flap without damaging the brain

GRAND ROUNDS – The practice of a department-wide meeting where cases are presented and discussed publicly for comment, criticism or suggestions for the approach to solving a diagnostic dilemma

HALLUCINOSIS – alcoholic hallucinosis (or alcohol-related psychosis) is a complication of withdrawal in alcoholics

HEMOSTASIS – Coagulating a bleeding blood vessel or placing a hemotatic clip on it

HEPATO-RENAL SYNDROME – A condition of physiologic stress when the function of the liver influences the renal function in a deleterious fashion causing fluid retention

HYPERKALEMIA – The potential threat of tissue damage in areas deprived of blood circulation as in both nutrition and oxygen supply

INTERSTICES – The potential spaces between each of the cells in the body

ISCHEMIC THREATENED – The potential threat of tissue damage in areas deprived of blood

ISMS – Illinois State Medical Society

KAYEXCELATE ENEMA – A chemical used as a per rectal enema that removes excess potassium from the blood

LIBRIUM – Sedative medication effective in managing seizures

MENINGES – Covering encasing the entire Central Nervous System

MUCOPURALENT – Purulent (pus) associated with infection

MYELOGRAM – A diagnostic study of the spinal fluid spaces of the brain and/or spinal cord with instillation of radio-opaque iodinated dye

NEUROANATOMY – Any aspect of the anatomy of the nervous system

NEUROPHYSIOLOGY – The scientific study of the functions of the nervous system

PATHOPHYSIOLOGY – The study of the diseases and disorders of the normal neurophysiology

PHLEBOTOMY – Action of drawing blood for analysis, testing etc.

PLATELET THROMBI – A clot within a blood vessel made up solely of platelets

PNEUMOCOCCAL – A specific type of infection, commonly pneumonia ,but pneumoncoccal bacteria can infect any tissue

PNEUOMOTHORAX – An air leak in the lung causing it to collapse and malfunction

# Where Do Doctors Hide Their Wings?

PUBIS – The anterior structure of the pelvis that forms the pubic bone

RESECTED – To surgically trim or excise

"SLEEP THE PATIENT" – Induction of anesthesia

THIAMINE – A vital vitamin for normal neural function. Its marked deficiency leads to an altered mental status

TERTIARY – Order, 3rd in place; functions are categorizes as primary, secondary or tertiary levels of importance

WHITE THROMBI – another name for platelet clots

XYPHOID – the lower most portion of the sternum

1600 - 1700 HOURS – 4:00 p.m. - 5:00 p.m.

*WHERE DO DOCTORS HIDE THEIR WINGS?* Is a collection of 27 short stories. As incredulous as some may seem, they are all true. Some chapters will have you laughing while others might make you cry. The book is a recap of the author's training as a PA and his first years in the field of medicine.

The author's mentors (doctors with wings) taught him to love their craft and to continually hunger for ever-expanding depths of knowledge. In his own words, "it was at their sides that I grew to love my patients as persons. They taught me how to distinguish the person from the malady, honoring the best in each of them so that they may, in turn, contribute to others."

This book is meant to start a conversation with patients saying to doctors, "show me your wings."

CPSIA information can be obtained at www.ICGtesting.com
Printed in the USA
LVOW08s0806140913

352354LV00003B/3/P